BEST MEALS FOR MUSCLE

This book is intended as a reference volume only, not as a medical manual.
The information given here is designed to help you make informed decisions about your health.
It is not intended as a substitute for any treatment that may have been prescribed by your doctor.
If you suspect that you have a medical problem, we urge you to seek competent medical help.

Mention of specific companies, organizations, or authorities in this book does not imply
endorsement by the author or publisher, nor does mention of specific companies, organizations,
or authorities imply that they endorse this book, its author, or the publisher.

Internet addresses and telephone numbers given in this book
were accurate at the time it went to press.

© 2020 by Hearst Magazines, Inc.

All rights reserved.
No part of this publication may be reproduced or transmitted in any form or by any means,
electronic or mechanical, including photocopying, recording, or any other
information storage and retrieval system, without the written permission of the publisher.

Men's Health is a registered trademark of Hearst Magazines, Inc.

Photographs by:
Jim White 4
Getty Images cover, back cover, 6, 10, 12, 14, 20, 24, 27-29, 31, 34, 37-38, 43-44, 46, 49-50, 53, 55-56, 59-60, 79, 82
Mike Garten 63, 65, 73, 84, 88, 113-115
Sam Kaplan 67
Ted and Chelsea Cavanaugh 69
Danielle Daly 71, 75, 97, 99, 117, 121, 125
Con Poulos 77, 105
Thomas MacDonald and Mitch Mandel 94
Michael Hedge 101
Chris Court 109

Book design by Laura White

Library of Congress Cataloging-in-Publication Data is on file with the publisher.

978-1-950099-64-1

2 4 6 8 10 9 7 5 3 1 paperback

HEARST

65+ Muscle-Building Meals and Snacks

BEST MEALS FOR MUSCLE

A NO-BULLSH*T 3-WEEK PLAN FOR BIG GAINS

By Jim White, R.D., and the editors of **Men's Health**

MH BEST MEALS FOR MUSCLE

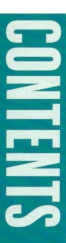

CONTENTS

4 INTRODUCTION

6 CHAPTER 1
What Makes Muscle

14 CHAPTER 2
Macros for Muscle Growth

24 CHAPTER 3
When to Eat

28 CHAPTER 4
The Science of Protein Supplements

34 CHAPTER 5
Master The Meal Plan
- **42** WEEK 1
- **48** WEEK 2
- **54** WEEK 3

60 MEAL PLAN RECIPES
- 62 BEAR-SIZED PB&J
- 64 HEARTY BEEF AND BEAN CHILI
- 66 TRIPLE DECKER CHICKEN CLUB
- 68 SALMON ARUGULA SALAD
- 70 CHICKEN MOLE TACOS
- 72 MUSTARD MAPLE PORK CHOPS
- 74 LIME TILAPIA WITH CITRUS-AVOCADO SALSA
- 76 SEARED SALMON WITH ROASTED CAULIFLOWER
- 78 SAUSAGE AND BROCCOLI RABE PASTA
- 80 ORANGE SWEET POTATO SALAD WITH CHICKEN
- 81 VEGETARIAN STIR-FRY

82 BONUS RECIPES

BREAKFASTS
- 83 SMOKED SALMON AND SCRAMBLED EGGS ON TOAST
- 84 BACON AND EGG FRIED RICE
- 86 RICOTTA AND LOX BREAKFAST BURRITO
- 87 BROCCOLI SPEARS OMELET
- 88 BEST-EVER SHAKSHUKA
- 90 SPINACH, EGG, AND CHEESE SANDWICH
- 91 GREEN EGGS AND HAM

LUNCHES
- 92 CHICKEN AVOCADO TACOS
- 93 SWEET ONION SALMON SALAD
- 94 TURKEY SLIDERS
- 96 JERK CHICKEN WITH CUCUMBER MANGO SALAD

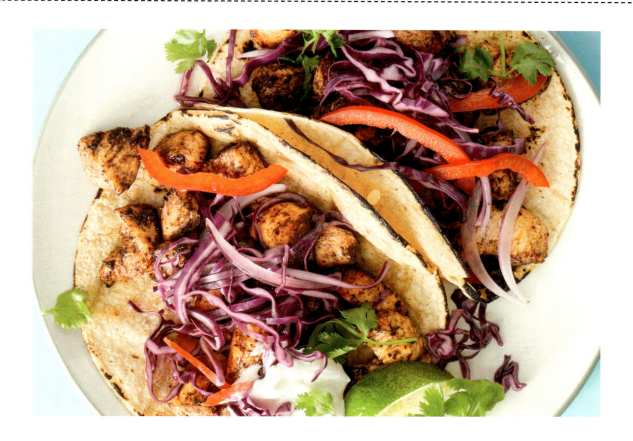

98	SALMON BLT WITH HERBED SPREAD
100	MISO EGGPLANT GRAIN BOWL
102	TUNA TACOS
103	CARNITAS BURRITO BOWL
104	SWEET AND STICKY TOFU
106	CHEESY BLACK BEANS AND GREENS

DINNERS
107	QUINOA-STUFFED BELL PEPPERS
108	POTSTICKER AND VEGETABLE STIR-FRY
110	SPICY PORK FAJITAS
111	SUNDRIED TOMATO AND FETA BAKED CHICKEN
112	PAPRIKA CHICKEN WITH CRISPY CHICKPEAS AND TOMATOES
114	HERBED MOJO STEAK AND CRISPY POTATOES
116	SHEET PAN CHICKPEA CHICKEN
118	CHILI MANGO CHICKEN
119	SWEET AND SOUR PORK
120	FRESH VEGGIE BEEF RAGU
122	SALMON TERIYAKI WITH ASPARAGUS
123	SMOKY AND SPICY SAUSAGE HEROES
124	SPICED MEATBALL PITAS WITH CRISPY COLE SLAW

Yep, this Chicken Mole Taco is what muscle is made of. More gains-boosting recipes start on page 60.

INTRODUCTION

This Changes Everything

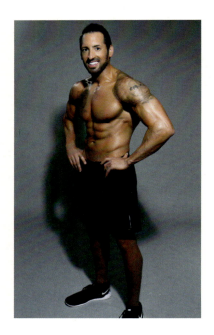

Jim White can divide his life into two eras: pre-gains and post-gains. That's how radically his world shifted when he started hitting the weight room.

Obviously there were the physical differences that distinguish the Jim White of today (an RDN, exercise physiologist, and owner of his own fitness and nutrition studio) from his former skinny self. He gained 70 pounds of lean muscle over the course of two years. He went from struggling to lift 65 pounds on the bar to bench-pressing 295. He's just plain jacked. But the biggest distinctions happened on another level.

"My whole life totally changed," says White. "Not only for my body, but for my sports. I was more aggressive. I played more. It led me to such a big place that I decided to make it my career to help hard-gainers build muscle and get to that next level."

Pre-gains Jim was not a pillar of health and fitness. Before he got serious at age 15 about packing on muscle, he ate, as he says, "like a bird." No fruits, no vegetables. He didn't consume enough calories, and what he did eat was mostly processed and loaded with sugar. He played baseball and basketball but stayed away from regular strength training.

"I was a skinny kid, so I was scared of the weight room," says White. "But I always wanted to be bigger, stronger, and faster."

So how did he end up going from 135 pounds to 195 pounds of muscle? He changed his diet. He bumped up his daily calorie intake to 3,500 and started eating six meals a day. Suddenly his energy skyrocketed, so extra time in the gym became easier. He gained confidence, too, which made 5 pounds more on the bar feel like less of a leap. Every day he got one step closer to his goals.

The right nutrition created the perfect storm for muscle growth. It gave White the energy to lift harder, and when he wasn't lifting, it gave him the perfect fuel for rebuilding his muscles bigger and stronger.

His new routine wasn't always easy. The spike in calorie intake meant he often ate when he wasn't hungry. "I had to focus on consistency and eat high-quality foods six times a day for two years. It took a lot of discipline and tenacity," says White. But the physical differences he quickly saw in his body kept him motivated.

White has since built upon and perfected the nutrition techniques he used in high school—combining the right foods, timing meals, and balancing macros to hit calorie quotas without feeling constantly full. He has shared his methods with thousands of clients, from athletes to beginners, helping them build big arms, six-pack abs, and tree-trunk legs. Here, he shares the foolproof strategy for kickstarting your gains so you can eat what you love as you add on lean, clean muscle.

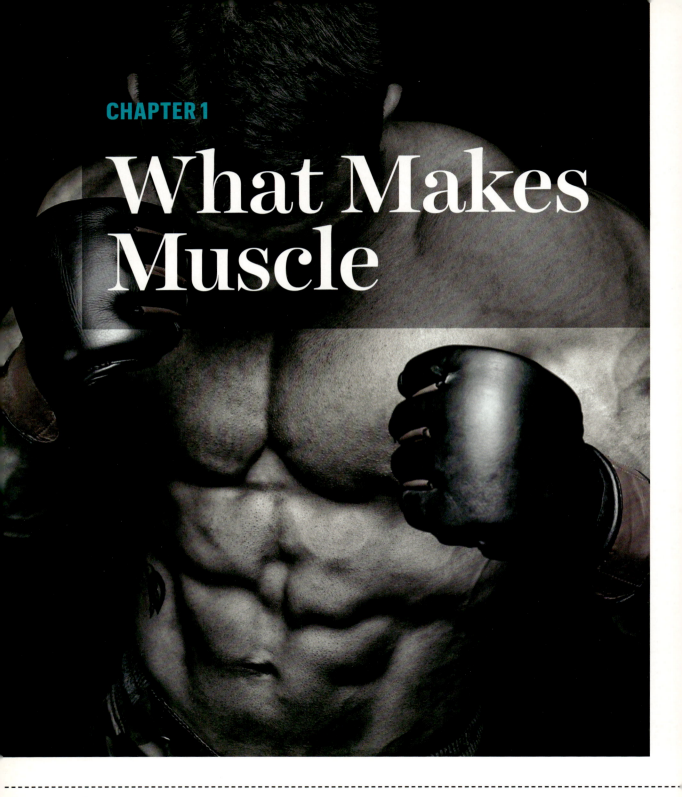

CHAPTER 1

What Makes Muscle

Building muscle is complex. It's about your workout, your nutrition, your hormones, your rest. The research can feel endless, and your feed of fit-fluencers claiming to know the secret can seem equally infinite. There's a ton to consider, and with so many potential paths to gains, cranking out bicep curls till your arms fall off may seem like the perfect move.

But the reality is that your muscles don't grow in the gym. The process of cells rushing to rebuild your torn-down muscle fiber happens when you rest. And what you eat when you're not pumping iron can mean the difference between packing on lean, clean muscle and destroying the very thing you hope to gain in the first place.

"Nutrition is the cornerstone to building lean muscle," says White. "If the protein isn't there, muscles won't grow. If the carbs aren't there, you feel sluggish. If the fat isn't there, energy levels and overall health suffer."

White's clients are a testament to the impact nutrition has on reaching your muscle goals. Take Evan, for example. Prior to working with White, his relationship with food was rocky. He didn't think it was possible to eat thousands of calories a day and remain lean and muscular. As for working out, he prioritized quantity over quality, clocking about 200 situps seven days a week. White got Evan on a 3,500-calorie meal plan. That meant eating six times a day and loading up on lean proteins, complex carbohydrates, and essential fats. Foods like eggs, avocado, and brown rice became Evan's daily staples. White also added variety to his workouts and built in rest days to promote recovery. In just three months on White's regimen, Evan gained 20 pounds of muscle.

"Once I embraced Jim's guidance on proper diet and exercise, I found myself getting bigger and stronger than I thought I could be," he says.

TOP 3 MUSCLE-MAKERS

When it comes to packing on muscle, White says these three factors should top your to-do list.

CONSISTENCY

Eat a consistent amount of food every day in order to maintain and maximize your muscle gains. If you down 4,000 calories on Sunday, but eat half that amount on Monday, your body won't have a constant fuel source and it'll slow down your growth. Follow a meal plan, prep as much food as possible, and stick with it.

PROTEIN

Anchor your plate with protein. It's the building block of muscle. Aim for around 30 grams at every meal, and make sure you get branched-chain amino acids (BCAAs), preferably from natural food sources. These are found in meat, fish, eggs, and nuts, among other foods, and are the essential amino acids to creating muscle.

CARBOHYDRATES

Hit your carb quota with every meal and snack. This is the key to fueling your muscles pre-workout and refueling them after. Without adequate glycogen (your body's stored form of carbs), you cannot expect your muscles to work to their full potential. Likewise, without adequate glycogen replenishment after workouts, you cannot expect proper muscle protein synthesis.

What Your Workout Does

Make no mistake, those squat and bent-over row supersets you've been hammering out are essential to the muscle-building process. It's just not the whole thing. In order for your muscles to grow, they need a good reason. To keep up with your habit of moving heavy objects is a good reason. To maintain that groove in your couch is not. Teach your muscles to expect stress and they'll work to develop a way to deal with it. So start a solid strength training routine. It doesn't have to be grueling, just consistent. White recommends a good rotation of compound movements, like squats and bench presses, in a format like this:

Elements of a Solid Muscle-Building Program

8 to 12 reps per set	3 or 4 sets per exercise	2 or 3 days per week

Be sure to get at least two minutes of rest between each set. Your muscles need time to recover between bursts. If you reach for the dumbbells after just 30 seconds, you likely won't be able to hit your reps with maximum strength. Every move during a resistance workout causes your muscles to undergo trauma. Churning out pushups or deadlifting a pair of dumbbells creates small tears in your muscle fiber. This triggers a response. Your muscles want to be more prepared for the next time they are called to perform. So they repair the tears, and end up stronger than they were before—*if* they have the right fuel (more on that later).

On a cellular level, it happens like this: Satellite cells—cells that live outside of your muscle fibers—rush to the rescue at the first signs of trauma. They multiply, then fuse to your muscle fiber, mending the tears and building your muscles back up bigger than when you started. Satellite cells do their best work with a mix of hormones and protein, which is exactly where the right nutrition comes into play.

BEST MEALS FOR MUSCLE | CHAPTER 1

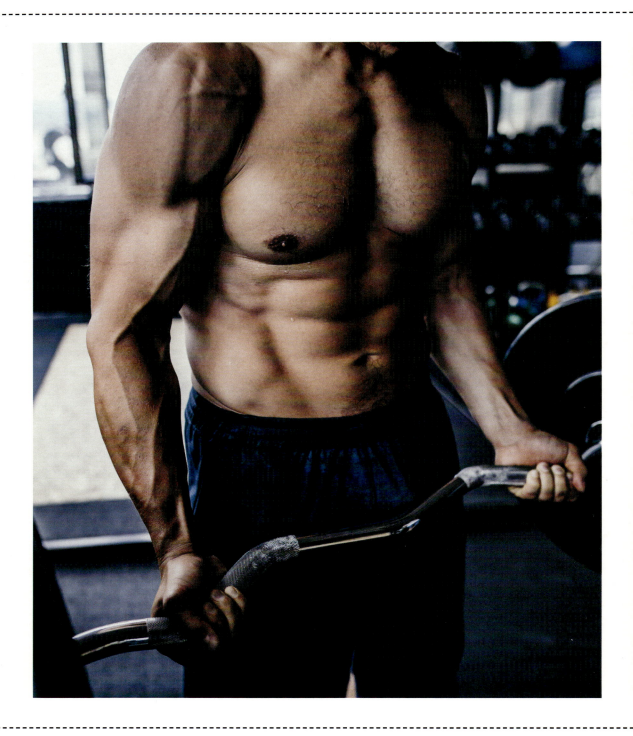

How Grub Becomes Gains

What you eat affects muscle growth in two main ways: It provides the protein that is used to build your new muscle, and it supports the biological processes that turn it into muscle. It would be easy to say that all you need to supercharge your gains is protein, protein, and more protein. But your body relies on more than one type of macro to convert food into muscle. Here's how it all (literally) breaks down.

PROTEIN

Studies show that consuming protein boosts the net balance of protein in your body and promotes muscle growth. Muscle cells are made of protein, which is why you need to eat enough of it if you want to pack on muscle. When you consume protein, your body breaks it down into components called amino acids. These amino chains are then used by satellite cells and your body's growth hormones as building blocks for muscle repair and growth after a workout. The process of protein breaking down and new protein being created is called protein turnover. For your muscles to get bigger, protein synthesis has to outpace protein breakdown. Resistance training breaks down protein, so to replace the protein that is broken you have to get it from food.

CARBOHYDRATE

If protein makes up the building blocks of muscle, carbs are the fuel. After you consume carbs, whether in a bagel or rice bowl, they're first broken down into glucose. What isn't immediately used is stored as glycogen. Your body relies on this stored form of carbohydrates to make it through a grueling workout and to support recovery afterward, so you need a solid supply. Eating carb-rich foods pre-workout increases glycogen stores by 42 percent, according to a study in the *Journal of Applied Physiology*. More glycogen means more energy to hoist that kettlebell overhead.

FAT

Fat helps grease the muscle-making wheels. Fat is critical to overall health, and in fact certain micronutrients can't be absorbed by the body unless fat is present in your diet. It also helps keep the hormone testosterone (a major muscle-building player) at optimal levels. Testosterone is derived from cholesterol. In order to support your "good" cholesterol (HDL), you need to eat healthy fats, such as those found in olive oil, avocados, and walnuts.

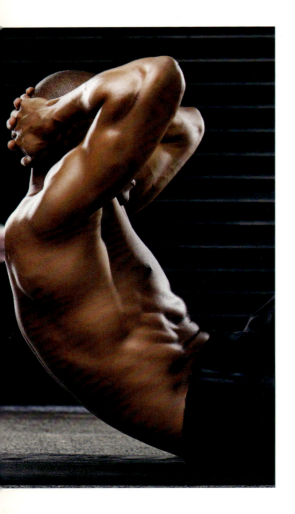

How to Power Up Your Hormones

Hormones are your body's messaging system, and they tell other parts of your body what to do, including make muscle. But they are touchy and can pretty easily get thrown out of whack. Disrupt your levels of cortisol (a.k.a. the stress hormone), for instance, and you may be more likely to store fat. To keep them in prime muscle-building balance there are essential things you must do: Eat enough calories, get enough sleep (to decrease cortisol levels), limit stress through practices like exercise and meditation, and allow for adequate rest from strength training exercises.

Although your entire arsenal of hormones plays a role in helping you reach your muscle goals, some have a bigger part than others. Here are some of the key players and how you can best support them.

INSULIN

Insulin sensitivity (how well your body responds to the release of insulin) has been shown to be positively correlated to muscle mass. When you eat carbohydrates, your body breaks them down into glucose. Insulin responds by transporting that glucose to your muscles. When your muscle cells open to accept the glucose, they are also able to accept amino acids and creatine, critical muscle-builders. Insulin also boosts protein synthesis.

▶ **SUPPORT IT:** For an optimal muscle-building environment, you want to keep your insulin levels steady throughout the day. Do this by eating six meals daily and watching your glycemic load. Foods with a low glycemic index (GI) take a while to digest, ensuring glucose slowly enters your bloodstream, instead of rapidly, which causes insulin spikes. But you don't need to stick to low GI foods. Smart combos, like those in White's meal plan, maintain an overall low glycemic load, so your insulin levels stay stable.

TESTOSTERONE

Testosterone is king when it comes to building muscle. It signals for the muscle-building process to commence, spurring satellite cells into action.

▶ **SUPPORT IT:** Good news: Lifting weights can help increase testosterone in the short term. For long-term support, keep your overall wellness in check by getting enough sleep, minimizing stress, and maintaining a healthy body weight.

GROWTH HORMONE AND IGF-1

Growth hormone and insulin-like growth factor 1 (IGF-1) go hand-in-hand. Growth hormone stimulates the production of IGF-1, which aids in repairing and building muscle.

▶ **SUPPORT IT:** Foods rich in melatonin, such as strawberries, walnuts, and eggs, can help boost the release of Human Growth Hormone (HGH).

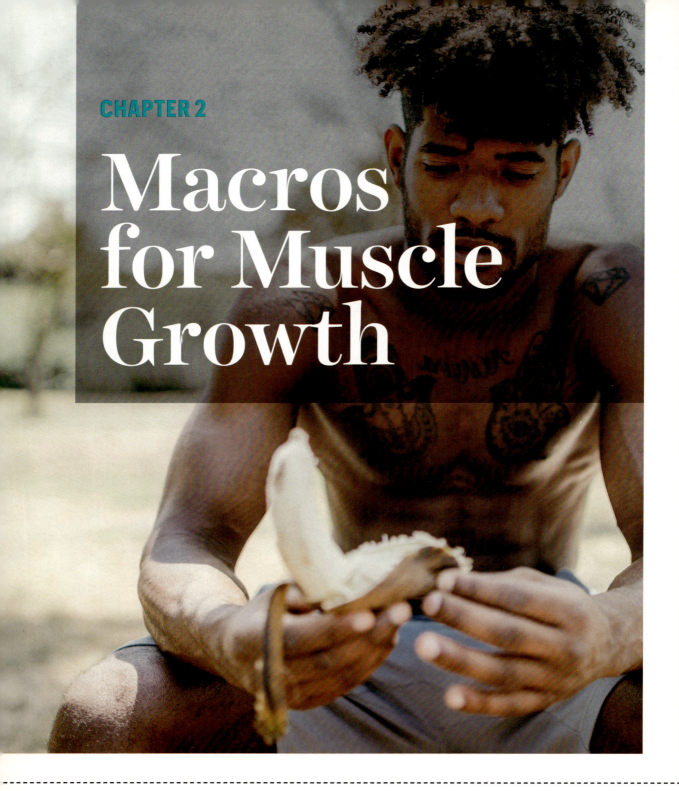

CHAPTER 2

Macros for Muscle Growth

Your body requires a diverse mix of nutrients to keep the engine humming. Those you need in large quantities are macronutrients. They consist of protein, carbohydrate, and fat. Those you need in small quantities are micronutrients, things like iron and vitamin C.

Macronutrients directly influence muscle growth. When you get your macro ratios down perfectly, expect to see your gains skyrocket. Why stick to ratios? On this plan, you'll be significantly increasing your calorie intake from your usual amount. If done incorrectly, you'll have a greater chance of gaining mostly body fat. If done the right way, you'll have a greater chance of gaining clean, lean muscle. Here's the optimal amount of protein, carbohydrate, and fat you should have on your plate to build muscle:

50 percent calories from carbohydrate | **25 percent calories from protein** | **25 percent calories from fat**

Don't stress if you don't hit your percentages exactly at every meal. Research shows it's more about the big picture. White suggests making these macros your overall daily goal and trying to stay within 5 percent over and under each number. (For example, your daily carbohydrate intake can vary between 45 percent and 55 percent.)

WHAT'S A MACRO WORTH?

Protein: 1 g = 4 calories

Carbohydrate: 1 g = 4 calories

Fat: 1 g = 9 calories

A MACRO-BALANCED PLATE

So what does a breakdown of 50 percent carbs, 25 percent protein, and 25 percent fat look like? Here are some quick and clean ideas to help you put it in context:*

4 egg whites
+ ¾ cup sweet potatoes
+ ¼ avocado

6 oz tofu
+ 1 cup brown rice
+ 10 asparagus spears
+ 2 Tbsp teriyaki sauce

3 oz deli turkey
+ 1 slice cheddar cheese
+ 2 slices whole grain bread
+ 1 apple

SMOOTHIE:
1 ¼ cups plain nonfat Greek yogurt
+ 2 Tbsp peanut butter
+ ½ cup strawberries
+ 1 banana

CHICKEN TACOS:
3 oz chicken breast
+ 2 corn tortillas
+ 1 cup beans and rice
+ ¼ avocado
+ 1 Tbsp hot sauce

*Macro ratios in these meal ideas are approximate.

Find Your Daily Calorie Intake

Before your macro numbers mean anything, you need to determine your optimal daily calorie intake. Eating the right amount of calories is crucial to bulking up. Eat too few and you'll burn through muscle. Eat too many of the unhealthy kind and you'll pack on fat.

Calories help fuel your workouts, so you're going to need a decent amount of them. Strength training burns a lot of calories, and those muscles your strength training creates burn calories even when you're at rest, according to studies. And muscle requires more maintenance than fat because it does more than fat and is denser than fat. All that maintenance requires calories. If your body can't find enough calories to make energy, it'll look to the muscle for fuel, breaking down the exact thing you just worked so hard to build.

"If you don't have the right fuel, you're not going to have the energy and protein to build muscle," says White.

However, eating too many empty calories won't help you hit your goals either. It is possible to gain muscle if you eat too many calories, but it's just more likely to come with a layer of fat. If you want quality lean muscle, you need to find your personal calorie sweet spot. Here's how:

FIND YOUR BASAL METABOLIC RATE (BMR)

Your BMR is how many calories you need to consume for your body to perform life-sustaining functions, like breathing.

Here's the formula:

66 + (6.2 x your desired weight in pounds) + (12.7 x your height in inches) − (6.76 x your age in years).

> It may sound complicated but stay with it. Say you're 35 and 6'1" and want to weigh 180 pounds; your BMR is 1,873.

MULTIPLY YOUR BMR BY YOUR ACTIVITY FACTOR

Now gauge your fitness:

LITTLE TO NO ACTIVITY (you rarely work out): **1.2**

MILDLY ACTIVE (you work out 1 or 2 times a week): **1.3**

MODERATELY ACTIVE (you work out 3 or 4 times a week): **1.4**

EXTREMELY ACTIVE (you go to the gym every day): **1.5**

The result is the number of daily calories you take in to reach your goal for your activity level. So for an inactive 35-year-old, that's 2,248 calories. If you become more active, just adjust the math.

From here, you can determine your personal macro intake for building muscle.

(Daily Calories x Macro Percentage) / Macro Calories Per Gram

For example: If you require 3,000 calories per day, here's how to calculate your macros:

PROTEIN	**CARBOHYDRATE**	**FAT**
(3,000 x 0.25) / 4 = 187.5 g protein per day	(3,000 x 0.50) / 4 = 375 g carbohydrate per day	(3,000 x 0.25) / 9 = 83 g fat per day

Why Macros Matter

Protein, carbohydrate, and fat all serve up some serious muscle-building benefits, but it's all about the balance.

PROTEIN

Piling your plate with protein provides your body with more resources to build muscle, keeps you full longer, and helps your body perform a range of other functions. But be careful of overdoing it. "The muscle-building capacity is around 30 grams of protein per meal," says White. "There isn't necessarily a huge additional muscle-building benefit to eating more. Plus, you're robbing yourself of other nutrients." Think of it like this: You could eat a six-egg omelet for breakfast and knock out a chunk of your daily protein goals, but that might not leave much room for other nutritional needs. You very likely may end up too full to pair those eggs with some energy-boosting carbs, and you might not be hungry enough later for the hearty lunch you need to eat to hit your calorie quota for the day.

STOCK UP ON: Eggs

Of all the protein sources you can eat, eggs have one of the highest biological values for protein. That basically means your body best absorbs and utilizes the protein in eggs to support muscle growth and other functions. On top of that, they're affordable and versatile. Hard-boil a dozen at the start of the week to have quick calorie boosters on hand. Grab some as a snack or smash one on a sandwich.

CARBOHYDRATE

Carbs give you the energy that you need to push more weight. Eat too few and you'll get confused, fatigued, irritable, and weak—not what you need to crush it at the gym. White recommends that 50 percent of your carb intake be from whole grains like oatmeal, whole wheat bread, and quinoa, which all provide a bigger nutritional bang for your buck than refined grains.

STOCK UP ON: Oatmeal

It can go savory or sweet, and you can doctor it up with whatever you have on hand. A serving of oatmeal is packed with the fiber essential for maintaining insulin levels throughout the day. Plus, you'll get B vitamins, a solid hit of protein, and, ultimately, it'll give you the glycogen you need to crush your next workout. "It's like putting high-octane fuel into your muscles," says White.

FAT

Fat can be clean. The majority of your meals should be low- to medium-fat, says White. So instead of skinless chicken breast, grab a thigh on occasion. At the end of the day, you need to put on weight, and smart fat choices will help you do so.

STOCK UP ON: Olive Oil

Olive oil is incredibly easy to work with. Whip it into a salad dressing. Slather your chicken breast with it. Roast your vegetables in it. Whatever you do with it, its monounsaturated fats can add the essential fats you need in your meal to help you achieve optimal wellness. It's even been shown to improve insulin sensitivity, according to a study in *Scientific Reports*. The better your body responds to insulin, the better it can use the glucose it carries with it to support muscle growth.

MH | **BEST MEALS FOR MUSCLE** | **CHAPTER 2**

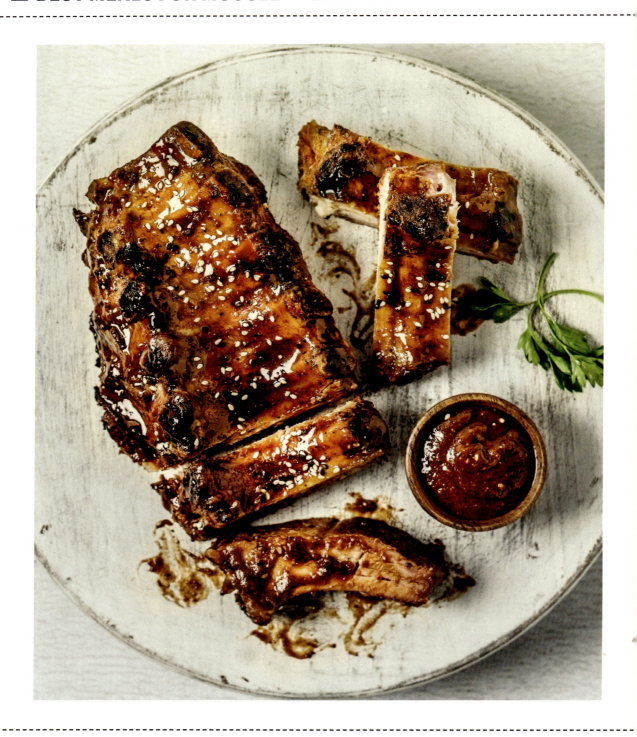

WHAT 30 GRAMS OF PROTEIN LOOKS LIKE

Not quite at your daily protein goal?
Grab one of these snacks, all of which provide around
30 g of protein, to quickly reach your ratios.

3 hard-boiled eggs + 1 cheese stick + 12 almonds	½ cup oats + 6 oz Greek yogurt + 2 Tbsp peanut butter	8 oz tofu + 1 cup broccoli + ½ cup brown rice
1 cup Greek yogurt + 2 Tbsp peanut butter	1 cup Greek yogurt + ½ cup granola	1 cup quinoa + 1 cup shelled edamame
1 cup cottage cheese + 23 almonds	1 cup liquid egg whites + ¼ cup shredded cheese	6 oz deli turkey + 1 slice cheese
2 eggs + 2 slices whole grain bread + 2 Tbsp peanut butter	4 oz sirloin 4 oz cooked chicken breast	2 protein waffles + 2 Tbsp peanut butter + 1 cup milk

Best Foods for Muscle Growth

There isn't one magic food for muscle growth. Ultimately, says White, a balanced diet containing essential fats, protein, complex carbohydrates, fruits, and vegetables is the best way to grow muscle. All of these provide different nutrients important to the body for proper metabolism. However, some pack more of a nutritional punch than others. Keep these in your weekly rotation:

BEST MEALS FOR MUSCLE | CHAPTER 2

Beef
Beef can be a lean source of rich protein and an excellent source of iron, which helps your muscles function.

Broccoli
Loaded with folate, and vitamins C and K, broccoli deserves more room on your dinner (or lunch) plate. Its high levels of vitamin C might even help cut down your post-workout recovery time. Vitamin C has been linked to shorter recovery times after intense workouts and less stiffness the day after, according to research in the *British Journal of Nutrition*.

Chicken
Chicken is an incredibly lean source of protein. A 3-ounce piece has 26 grams of protein and 3 grams of fat. There are countless ways to cook it, so it's easy to work into any meal plan.

Eggs
Eggs have a high biological value, provide a solid serving of protein, are rich in choline (which helps metabolize fat), and the list goes on. Eggs are insanely versatile, affordable, and effective at promoting muscle growth.

Greek Yogurt
One cup of Greek yogurt will net you around 15 to 20 grams of protein. Plus, it's an excellent source of calcium and vitamin D. Increased levels of vitamin D have been shown to boost athletic performance, according to a study published in the *Journal of Sports Sciences*. Just watch out for flavored varieties, which are often loaded with sugar.

Milk
No, it's not as trendy as your oat and almond options, but one serving of milk will give you around 8 grams of protein and a solid dose of calcium and vitamin D. What takes

it to the next level, however, is its fat content, which promotes absorption of vitamin D. Pour a glass with your next meal.

Oatmeal

The energy boost alone is enough to warrant a mention of this hearty grain. But oatmeal does more than power you through your leg-day burner. It's also rich in fiber, which can help you avoid insulin spikes.

Salmon

Lean protein? Check. Omega-3 fatty acids? Yep. This fatty fish also helps prevent inflammation and protects your heart.

Sweet Potatoes

These are rich in vitamin C and fiber and are an excellent source of carbohydrate for lasting energy. Prepare like you would a classic baked potato, or chop and roast as the side to the protein of your choice.

Walnuts

Walnuts are rich in essential fatty acids and antioxidants. They also have more omega-3 fatty acids than any other nut, which may help improve your HDL (healthy) cholesterol.

Foods to Avoid in Excess

Watch your intake of empty calories. These are foods that don't provide a significant source of nutrients, don't fill you up, and are typically loaded with the stuff that will lead to dirty gains (read: tons of sugar). You don't need to completely cut these out of your life, just enjoy in moderation.

**Alcohol | Candy | Cookies | Doughnuts | Energy Drinks
Fried Foods | Potato Chips | Soft Drinks | High-Sugar Coffee Drinks**

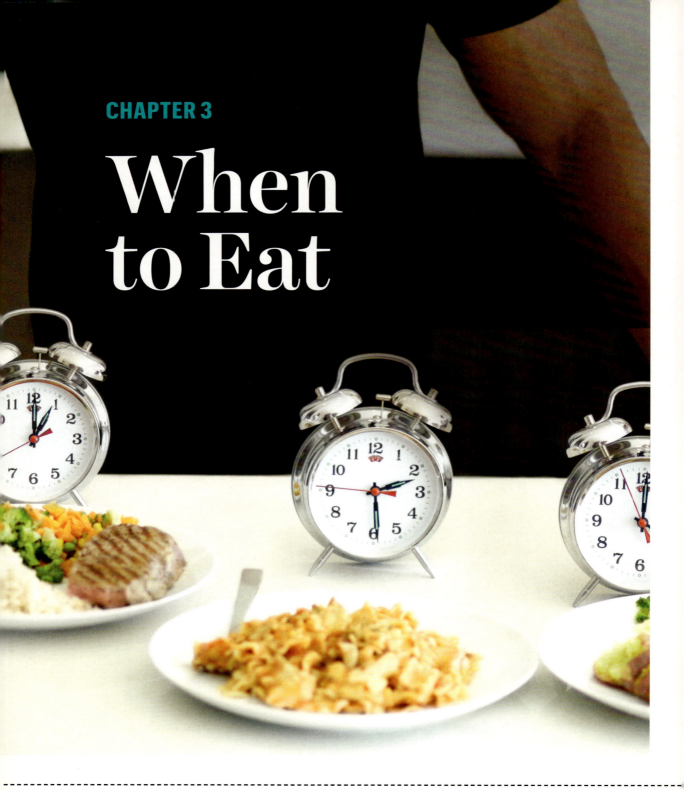

CHAPTER 3
When to Eat

The timing of your meals and snacks is just as important as what you eat. Give your body the right fuel when it needs it and every single calorie in that turkey sandwich will be well used. Ultimately, you need to keep your meals in pace with your body. Your body can't properly digest 3,000 calories at once, so you have to space them out. But how do you decide when to start eating, when to stop, and when to add snacks? Follow these guidelines from White to make the most of every meal:

Eat 6 Times a Day

On this plan you will eat around 3,000 calories a day—some days more, some days less. If you break that down into your standard three-meals-a-day structure, that's 1,000 calories per meal. You might be able to eat that much, but you'll likely end up feeling sluggish and experience blood sugar ups and downs. Spacing your food intake across 3 meals and 3 snacks ensures you're not overwhelming your body.

Eat (Roughly) Every 3 Hours

Your body is constantly in a state of protein turnover, the process of protein being broken down and created. Eating the right foods gives the protein creation part of this process a major boost that lasts for three hours. Eat every 3 hours and you'll keep your body in a constant muscle-building mode. It'll also help keep your insulin levels stable.

Eat Within 1 Hour of Waking

You're going to want to start working on hitting your calorie goals pretty early in the day so you can space them out appropriately. Again, you want to avoid trying to down them all in one 3,000-calorie feast. Try to eat your first meal during your first hour out of bed.

Eat Your Last Meal at Least 3 Hours Before Bed

Eat any later than that and it can start to impact your sleep (a.k.a. your recovery zone). Give your body enough time to process everything before hitting the hay.

Best Meals for Muscle | Chapter 3

Timing Pre-Workout and Post-Workout

What you eat before a workout fuels how much weight you can lift (and the potential for muscle growth). What you eat after a workout fuels your muscle growth. Use these strategies from White to time them both just right.

Pre-Workout

TIME IT: 30 minutes to 3 hours pre-workout
MAKE IT: A combo of protein and carbohydrates

Why such a wide time range? Anything you down 3 hours to 30 minutes before hitting the weights will be your fuel. Tailor your plate to the length of time until you'll work out. If it's 2 to 3 hours, you can have a more substantial meal (like a turkey sandwich with fruit and whole grain crackers). "As you get into that 30- to 90-minute window, you want fast-digesting food, like yogurt with granola and nuts," says White. "It's really a personal preference. Some people get GI distress if they eat before working out." Keep tweaking your timing until you find what makes you feel most energized.

Post-Workout

TIME IT: 1 hour post-workout
MAKE IT: A combo of protein and carbohydrates

After a workout, your muscles are in an optimal state to absorb carbohydrates. Once you put down the weights, your muscles start rebuilding the muscle fibers torn during your gym session. Give your muscles what they need to do this job and they will do it. White recommends eating 3 to 4 grams of carbs for every 1 gram of protein you consume. So if you eat 25 grams of protein, pair it with 75 to 100 grams of carbs. Protein will spark muscle synthesis, and carbs will restore the glycogen you used during your workout. Try this combo: 1 cup Greek yogurt for protein with ¾ cup granola, a small banana and 1 cup strawberries for a hit of nutrient-packed carbs.

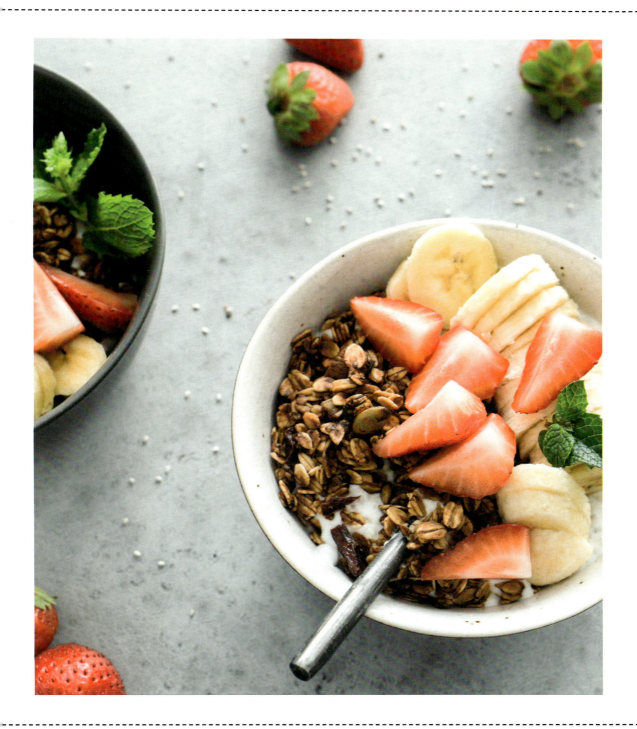

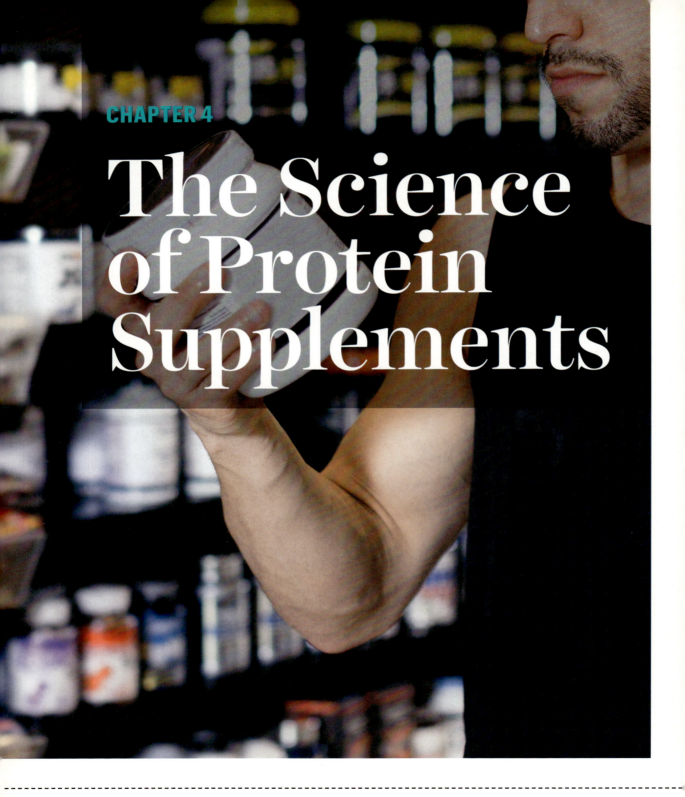

CHAPTER 4

The Science of Protein Supplements

Recently, it seems more and more foods are slapped with a "protein-packed" label. You can get your protein supplement in the form of powders, bars, ready-made shakes, cookies, and even pizza. It's incredibly convenient, but for optimal muscle growth you should get your protein from whole foods whenever possible. Here are three big reasons:

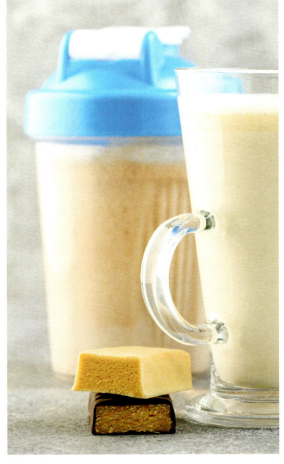

LESS PROCESSED: As powders are made, extras are mixed in—sodium, saturated fats, sugar. These things, in excess, aren't great for overall health. The beauty of whole foods? You know nothing's added.

NUTRIENT DENSE: Consider this: In addition to protein, an egg packs iron, vitamins, minerals, and carotenoids. Most supplements focus singularly on protein. Whole foods give you the bigger picture.

ADDITIVE-FREE: Protein supplements are laden with preservatives and flavoring agents that may cause digestive issues.

Also, don't forget the importance of good old-fashioned chewing. The biting and grinding process triggers enzymes in your stomach that help your body use what you eat for energy.

Complete Proteins

When it comes to building muscle, judge your protein on the content of its essential amino acids. Calories and taste are important too, but aminos should be the deal-breaker. Living tissue is made up of 22 different amino acids. Your body can make 13 of them. The other nine must come from food. If a particular food contains all nine amino acids, it's a complete protein.

Complete proteins are found in animal products, including all red meat, fish, poultry, pork, cheese, milk, and yogurt, as well as some plant-based foods. Add these to your grocery list:

WHOLE FOOD COMPLETE PROTEIN SOURCES

Food	Protein	Serving Size
Salmon	40 g	0.5 fillet
Chicken (skinless, boneless breast)	31 g	3.5 oz
Cottage cheese	24 g	1 cup
Quinoa	8 g	1 cup (cooked)
Eggs	8 g	1 egg
Tofu	8 g	3 oz
Swiss cheese	7 g	1 oz

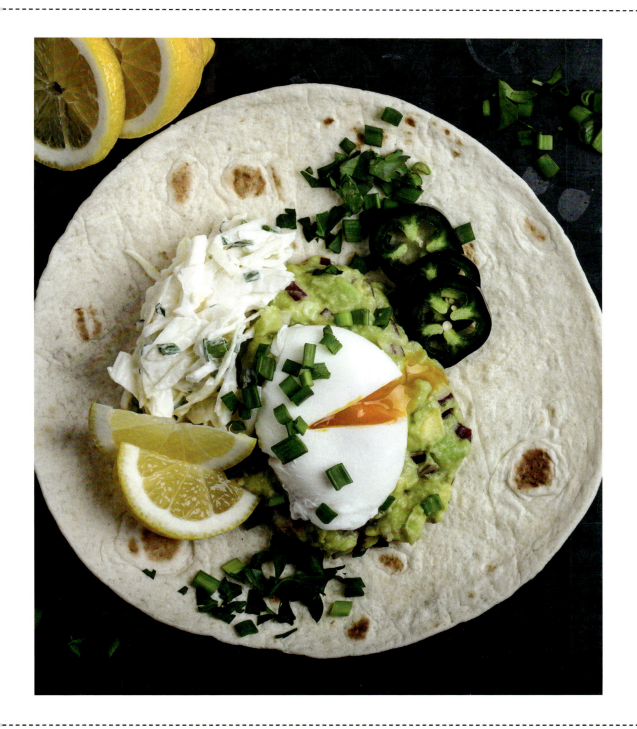

You can (and should) eat more than these proteins to fuel your muscle growth. You can trick your body into processing lots of foods as complete proteins, if you pair them with the right stuff. Try these satisfying pairings, all of which count as complete proteins:

| 1 slice whole grain bread + 2 Tbsp peanut butter | ½ cup rice + ½ cup black beans | ¼ cup hummus + 1 whole grain pita bread | ½ cup edamame + ½ cup quinoa |

If You Must Supplement, Do It Like This

Busy days happen. If you have to choose between downing a protein shake or nothing at all, choose the shake. But choose the right one. Here's how:

LOOK FOR THE SEAL. Protein powders don't need FDA approval to hit the shelves, which means what you see isn't always what you get. Stick to brands stamped with a third-party certification, such as NSF Certified for Sport or U.S. Pharmacopeia.

PICK YOUR PROTEIN SOURCE. Most bars and powders will tell you its main protein source right in the name. If it doesn't, check the ingredients list. There are a ton of ways you can compare the quality of your protein source, but the big ones are dietary needs (i.e., you're allergic to or avoiding dairy), protein digestibility corrected amino acid score (PDCAAS), and digestible indispensable amino acid score (DIAAS). These two scores are measures of how well your body is able to digest and break down the protein in a given powder. The higher the score, the more essential amino acids your body is absorbing per unit of protein. Ultimately, whey is going to give you the most bang for your buck, says White. "Whey serves as the most impactful and cost-effective protein supplement," he says. "Where pea protein would be sufficient is for someone who cannot tolerate whey or casein, or prefers a plant-based diet."

PROTEIN SUPPLEMENT BREAKDOWN

Protein	What It's Made From	PDCAAS	DIAAS
Whey	Milk	1	109%
Casein	Milk	1	91.5%
Soy	Dehydrated soybean flakes	1	118%
Pea	Yellow peas	0.82	82%

FIND THESE THREE NUTRIENTS. A solid protein supplement contains BCAAs, which include three main muscle-building amino acids: leucine, isoleucine, and valine. They are typically listed on the nutrition label. White recommends products with a ratio of 2 parts leucine to 1 part isoleucine to 1 part valine.

MAKE SURE THERE ARE NONE OF THESE. A lot of muscle-sabotaging ingredients end up in protein supplements. Watch out for artificial sweeteners, like xylitol and sorbitol, which can mess with your digestion. Use unsweetened supplements instead. If you need a boost of flavor, add a bit of cinnamon or cocoa to your powders. Real sugar is fine, but look for less than 5 grams per serving to stay within the American Heart Association's recommended max of 36 grams of added sugar daily.

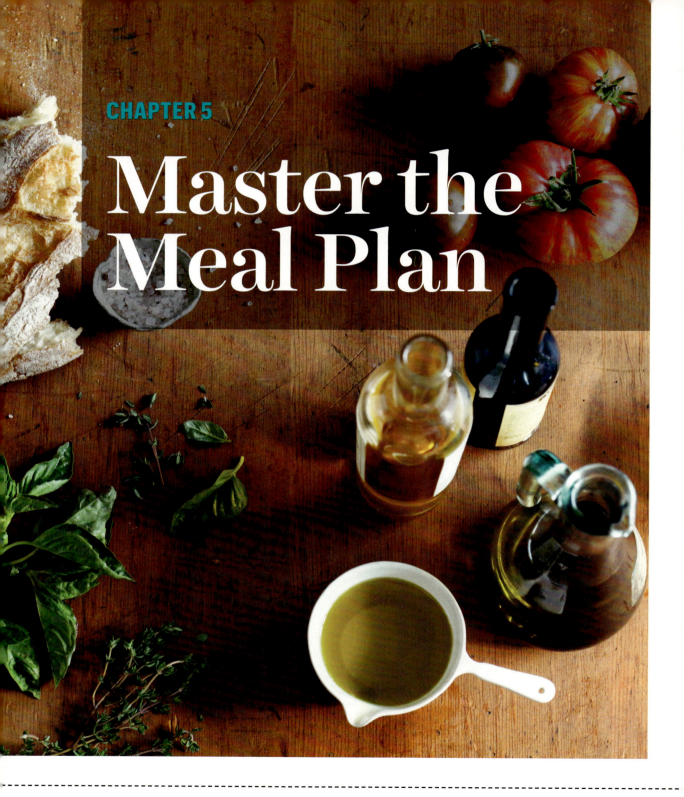

CHAPTER 5

Master the Meal Plan

This meal plan is your muscle-building foundation. White created it for maximizing muscle growth and minimizing effort in the kitchen. Every day of this plan provides the perfect macro mix to power you through your warm-up straight through to your most challenging finisher. This plan is ideal for beginners. Be sure to reassess your nutrition whenever you change your training goals.

It'll get you the results you want as it is, but can also be customized. Any time you want a little change, follow these guidelines.

MAKE IT YOURS

Eat in Any Order

If "brinner" is more your thing, go ahead and swap your breakfast with your dinner. Or your lunch with your dinner. Or breakfast with lunch.

Same Goes for Snacks

All snacks are interchangeable, so grab whatever you're craving.

Repeat Favorites

You can even eat the same meal every day, but White recommends switching things up to avoid boredom and ensure you're getting a full spectrum of nutrients.

Swap Out Proteins

You can replace any of the proteins with whatever your go-to is. That turkey sandwich can be a ham sandwich or a Tofurky sandwich. Just try to keep it close to gram for gram the same amount of protein.

Switch Up Sauces

White recommends meal prepping different sauces to add a hit of flavor to your proteins. Try cooking up three varieties of chicken breast—honey mustard, barbecue, and chipotle. Feel free to also kick things up with condiments like ranch, hot sauce, or salsa.

Do Dairy-Free Right

If you're lactose-intolerant, switch out any dairy ingredients with lactose-free versions. You'll get comparable calcium and other nutrients.

SUPERCHARGE YOUR GAINS WITH THESE

Water

Basic, but effective. Weight trainers who experienced dehydration before working out had lower one-repetition maximums than when they were hydrated, according to a *Journal of Strength and Conditioning* study. Plus, water can help decrease muscle soreness, speed up recovery, and keep your body's vital functions humming along so it can focus more on building muscle. How much water you need depends on a lot of factors, but aim for half your weight in ounces, says White. So, if you're 150 pounds, drink 75 ounces a day.

Fiber

Aim for 35 to 38 grams of fiber per day, says White. Fiber helps fill you up, regulate digestion, and control insulin levels.

Sleep

Remember, rest is where the magic happens. If you're in your 20s or 30s, try to get 7.5 hours to 8 hours to best support the muscle-making process. "Your body is preparing at night for muscle growth," says White. Not an asleep-in-60-seconds kind of person? White recommends avoiding eating and exercising three hours before bed and putting down electronics one to two hours before.

Meditation

Or any form of stress-relief. Stress causes your body to pump out cortisol. Too much cortisol increases body fat. Not the process you want to encourage when you're upping your calorie intake.

Electrolytes

Electrolytes help your muscles contract. When you work out, you lose electrolytes. Not enough electrolytes equals major muscle cramps. Don't let this interrupt your pump. Fuel up with electrolyte-rich foods before your workout, like bananas, Greek yogurt, or sports drinks (just watch out for a ton of added sugar).

CHECK YOUR PROGRESS (AND ADJUST ACCORDINGLY)

Packing on muscle takes time. But you might find that you need more calories to gain weight than the amount in the meal plan. If that's the case, try adding a couple of hundred more calories each day and see how your body responds. The easiest way to do this? With fat. Remember, fat provides 9 calories per gram, while carbohydrates and protein serve up just 4 calories per gram. You'll be able to layer on calories without getting too full. White suggests upping the olive oil in any of the recipes (1 Tbsp = 120 calories), adding some avocado as a side (½ avocado = 160 calories), or a good old-fashioned scoop of peanut butter (2 Tbsp = 190 calories).

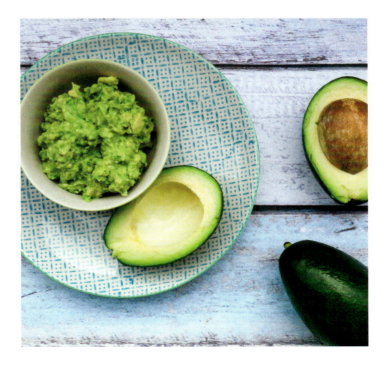

You can also bump up the calories by increasing your portions of carbs and veggies. A ½ cup of rice and 1 cup vegetables will net you about 150 calories. A ½ cup of beans weighs in at about 115 calories and provides a boost of fiber and protein.

BEST MEALS FOR MUSCLE | CHAPTER 5

How the Plan Works

This is a no-bull meal plan. Jim White designed it to provide efficiency and flexibility. You will not find complicated recipes or time-consuming cooking methods. Most of the meals here take about 15 minutes to prepare. And with our meal prep tips, you'll knock out the hard work all at once and eat clean all week.

These meals are also efficient in ingredients. You don't need to purchase cartloads of food each week, and you'll use all (or nearly all) of what you buy. We've built recipes around workhorse ingredients that'll get you to your macro goals without requiring a culinary degree. Every meal and snack bolsters your body's muscle-building processes.

If you want more variety, swap in any of the approved recipe variations and cooking methods in this section.

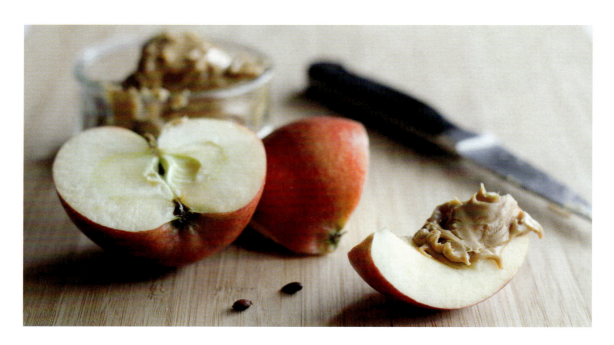

RECIPE POSSIBILITIES

Trail Mix Variations

¼ cup low-sugar granola
2 Tbsp pumpkin seeds
2 Tbsp pecans
2 Tbsp raisins

¼ cup low-sugar granola
2 Tbsp cashews
2 Tbsp unsweetened shredded coconut
2 Tbsp dried cranberries

¼ cup low-sugar granola
2 Tbsp slivered almonds
2 Tbsp walnuts
2 Tbsp raisins

Loaded English Muffin Variations

1 whole wheat English muffin
2 Tbsp peanut butter
½ sliced banana
1 Tbsp coconut flakes

1 whole wheat English muffin
2 Tbsp almond butter
¼ cup blackberries
1 Tbsp chia seeds

1 whole wheat English muffin
2 Tbsp peanut butter
¼ cup sliced strawberries
1 Tbsp coconut flakes

Cottage Cheese Protein Bowl Variations

1 ½ cups cottage cheese
2 cups pineapple
4 medium figs (sliced)
2 Tbsp walnuts

1 ½ cups cottage cheese
¼ avocado
1 cup cherry tomatoes
1 tsp hot sauce

1 ½ cups cottage cheese
¼ cup black beans
2 Tbsp salsa
cilantro

Apple and Almond Butter Variations

1 apple
2 Tbsp peanut butter
1 banana

2 Tbsp peanut butter
2 stalks celery

2 Tbsp peanut butter
¼ cup raisins

Cooking Methods

Unless otherwise noted, feel free to cook your proteins and vegetables using whatever method you prefer. Each meal and snack on this plan is portioned to keep you within your calorie goals, so you'll want to avoid any preparation that jacks up the calorie count, such as deep frying. Keep calorie additions within 100 calories, which is about 2 ½ teaspoons of olive oil. Here are some easy, yet delicious ways to make these meal-plan staples.

Proteins

You can grill, sauté, broil, or bake your meats and proteins. Use a maximum of 100 calories of your favorite fat (such as butter or olive oil).

CHICKEN *Basic Technique:* Preheat the oven to 350°F and bake the chicken breast for 20 to 25 minutes, or until an internal roasting thermometer reaches 170°F.

SALMON *Basic Technique:* Coat a medium skillet with cooking spray and set over high heat. Lightly coat the salmon with cooking spray. Add the salmon to the skillet and cook for 3 minutes on each side, or until the fish flakes easily. Check by cutting into the fillet.

STEAK *Basic Technique:* Heat a cast-iron skillet on high. Season steak with salt, pepper, and other seasonings as desired. Add 1 tablespoon of canola oil to the pan. Add the steak and sear, flipping every minute, for a total of about 6 minutes for medium rare.

Vegetables

Roasting is one of the easiest ways to cook vegetables. Just drizzle with olive oil and put in the oven. A good rule of thumb: 1 tablespoon of oil for every 2 pounds of vegetables. Follow these guidelines for some of White's go-to vegetables.

VEGETABLE ROASTING CHEAT SHEET

ASPARAGUS, 2 POUNDS

How to Cut: Snap off woody stems.
Roasting Time at 450°F: 10 to 15 minutes

BROCCOLI, 2 POUNDS

How to Cut: Trim and peel stems; split florets into 1½- to 2-in.-wide pieces.
Roasting Time at 450°F: 10 to 15 minutes

GREEN BEANS, 2 POUNDS

How to Cut: Trim stem ends.
Roasting Time at 450°F: 20 to 30 minutes

POTATOES, 2 POUNDS, UNPEELED

How to Cut: Slice into 2-in. pieces
Roasting Time at 450°F: 45 minutes

SWEET POTATOES, 2 POUNDS

How to Cut: Slice crosswise in half, then lengthwise into 1-in. wedges.
Roasting Time at 450°F: 30 minutes

SERVINGS

Unless otherwise noted, eat 1 serving of each meal or snack. Some recipes will require you to make multiple servings so you can save leftovers and eat them on another day, as indicated in the plan.

BEST MEALS FOR MUSCLE | WEEK 1

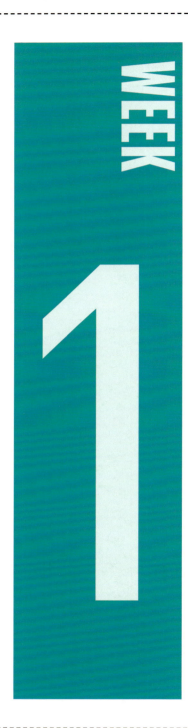

Shopping List

MEATS & PROTEINS

½ lb lean **GROUND BEEF**
1 dozen **EGGS**
8 oz **CHICKEN BREAST**
1 small **ROTISSERIE CHICKEN**
1 (6-oz) lean **PORK CHOP**
2 (5-oz) fillets **SALMON**
5 oz **SIRLOIN STEAK**
1 (12-oz) block **TOFU**
1 (12-oz) package **TURKEY BACON**
1½ lb low sodium **TURKEY DELI MEAT**
1 box high-protein **FROZEN WAFFLES**, such as Kodiak

DAIRY

¼ lb **CHEDDAR CHEESE**
7 oz **CHEESE** of your choice
2 (24-oz) containers **PLAIN COTTAGE CHEESE**
1 oz crumbled **FETA CHEESE**
1 (4-oz) package **GOAT CHEESE**
¼ lb **SWISS CHEESE**
1 (8-oz) jar **MAYO**
½ gallon **WHOLE MILK**
1 (32-oz) container plain full-fat **YOGURT**
2 (5.3 oz) servings full-fat **GREEK YOGURT**

PRODUCE

6 **APPLES**
1 (5-oz) container **ARUGULA**
1 bunch **ASPARAGUS**
2 medium **AVOCADOS**
5 **BANANAS**
2 cups **GREEN BEANS**
About 1 lb **BERRIES** of your choice
2 small heads **BROCCOLI**
2 **CARROTS**
1 head **GARLIC**
½ cup **GRAPES**
1 **LEMON**
2 leaves **LETTUCE**
1 (8-oz) package **MUSHROOMS**
1 **ONION**
½ **YELLOW ONION**
3 small **ORANGES**
1 **BELL PEPPER**
2 **PINEAPPLES**
1 (1½-lb) bag **BABY POTATOES**
2 **POTATOES**
2 **SWEET POTATOES**
1 bunch **SPINACH**
1 (16-oz) container **STRAWBERRIES**
2 **TOMATOES**

PANTRY

1 (6.3-oz) bag ALMONDS
1 (16-oz) jar natural ALMOND BUTTER
1 small jar DRIED BASIL
1 (15-oz) can CANNELLINI BEANS
1 (15-oz) can GARBANZO BEANS
1 (1-oz) package CASHEWS
1 small jar CHILI POWDER
1 (12-oz) bag DARK CHOCOLATE CHIPS
1 (12-oz) bag UNSWEETENED COCONUT FLAKES
COOKING SPRAY
1 (6-oz) package DRIED CRANBERRIES
1 small jar GROUND CUMIN
1 (16-oz) package GROUND FLAXSEED
1 (1-in.) piece GINGER
1 (12-oz) package GRANOLA
1 (8-oz) jar MUSTARD
1 small bottle OLIVE OIL
1 (6-oz) can PITTED GREEN OLIVES
1 (16-oz) jar NATURAL PEANUT BUTTER
1 (6-oz) jar prepared PESTO
1 (16-oz) bag PRETZELS
1 small jar RED PEPPER FLAKES
1 (13-oz) bag QUINOA
1 small jar DRIED ROSEMARY
SALT and PEPPER
1 small bottle LOW-SODIUM SOY SAUCE
1 small jar DRIED THYME

1 (3-oz) bag dry-packed SUN-DRIED TOMATOES
1 small bottle BALSAMIC VINEGAR
1 small bottle RED WINE VINEGAR
1 oz WALNUTS
1 (8.5-oz) box WHOLE GRAIN CRACKERS, such as Triscuits
2 WHOLE WHEAT BAGELS
1 loaf sliced WHOLE WHEAT BREAD
1 package WHOLE WHEAT ENGLISH MUFFINS
1 package WHOLE WHEAT 8-IN. TORTILLAS

MEAL PREP

Store all items in air-tight containers. If perishable, keep in your refrigerator.

ON DAY BEFORE STARTING MEAL PLAN

Cube 4 cups pineapple.

Cook 1⅔ cups quinoa according to package directions.

Cook 8 oz chicken breast.

Prep 3 servings Trail Mix (p. 45).

Dice 1 cup sweet potatoes.

ON DAY 3

Cube 4 cups pineapple.
Dice 1 cup sweet potatoes.
Slice ½ bell pepper.
Dice 1½ cups potatoes.
Slice 1 cup strawberries.

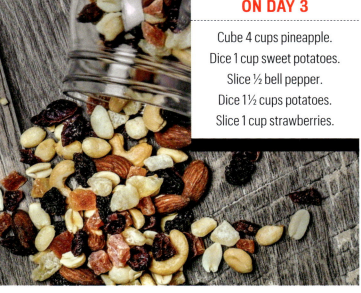

BEST MEALS FOR MUSCLE | WEEK 1

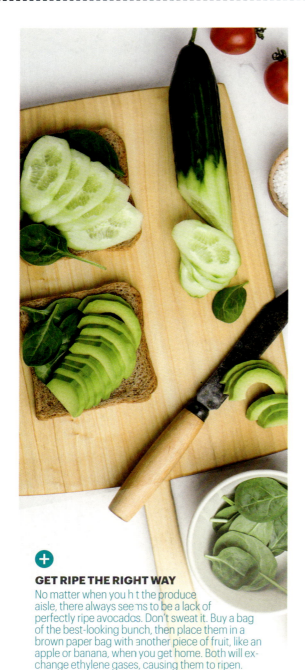

GET RIPE THE RIGHT WAY
No matter when you hit the produce aisle, there always seems to be a lack of perfectly ripe avocados. Don't sweat it. Buy a bag of the best-looking bunch, then place them in a brown paper bag with another piece of fruit, like an apple or banana, when you get home. Both will exchange ethylene gases, causing them to ripen.

DAY 1

Breakfast BAGEL AND YOGURT
Toast 1 whole wheat bagel and top with 1½ Tbsp peanut butter and 1 sliced banana. Eat with 1 5.3-oz serving plain full-fat Greek yogurt.

Snack COTTAGE CHEESE PROTEIN BOWL
Top 1½ cups plain cottage cheese with 2 cups cubed pineapple and 2 Tbsp ground flaxseed.

Lunch TURKEY SANDWICH
Toast 2 slices whole wheat bread and fill with 1 Tbsp sliced avocado, 6 oz low-sodium deli-sliced turkey, 1 slice Swiss cheese, a handful of spinach, and 1-2 slices each of onion and tomato. Eat with 1 small orange, 13 pretzels, and 1 cup whole milk.

Snack CHEESE, CRACKERS, FRUIT, AND NUTS
Eat 1 oz cheese of your choice, 6 whole grain crackers, 1 apple, and 24 almonds.

Dinner PORK CHOP AND QUINOA
Cook 6 oz lean pork chop and season as desired. Serve with ⅔ cup cooked quinoa and 1 cup broccoli roasted with 1 Tbsp olive oil.

Snack BANANA, PB, AND PRETZELS
Eat 1 sliced banana topped with 2 Tbsp natural peanut butter, and 13 pretzels.

NUTRITION (PER DAY): 3,587 CALORIES | 216 G PROTEIN | 378 G CARBOHYDRATES (51 G FIBER) | 146 G FAT

DAY 2

Breakfast BEAR-SIZED PB&J (p. 62)

Snack LOADED ENGLISH MUFFIN

Toast 1 whole wheat English muffin and fill with 2 Tbsp natural almond butter, 2 Tbsp dried cranberries, and 1 Tbsp unsweetened coconut flakes.

Lunch MEDITERRANEAN GRAIN BOWL

Preheat oven to 400°F. Cut 8 asparagus spears into 2-in. pieces. Place on rimmed baking sheet and toss with 1 Tbsp olive oil, salt, and pepper. Roast until soft and lightly brown, about 10 minutes. Combine 1 cup cooked quinoa with roasted asparagus, 1 oz crumbled feta cheese, 2 Tbsp pitted and chopped green olives, 2 Tbsp chopped sundried tomatoes, 1 Tbsp balsamic vinegar, 8 oz cooked chopped chicken breast, and half a 15-oz can garbanzo beans, rinsed and drained. Makes 2 servings. Refrigerate leftovers for Day 3 dinner.

Snack TRAIL MIX

Combine ¼ cup low-sugar granola with 6 cashews, 6 almonds, 4 walnut halves, and 1 Tbsp dark chocolate chips.

➕ **Tip:** When choosing a granola, stick to a max of 10 g of sugar per serving.

Dinner HEARTY BEEF AND BEAN CHILI (p. 64)

Refrigerate remaining for Day 3 lunch.

Snack APPLE AND ALMOND BUTTER

Slice 1 apple and dip in 2 Tbsp natural almond butter. Enjoy with 1 cup whole milk.

NUTRITION (PER DAY): 3,446 CALORIES | 193 G PROTEIN
307 G CARBOHYDRATES (64 G FIBER) | 171 G FAT

DAY 3

Breakfast SWEET POTATO HASH BOWL

Preheat oven to 425°F. On rimmed baking sheet, toss 1 cup diced sweet potatoes with 1 tsp olive oil, salt, and pepper. Bake until potatoes are crispy and fork tender, about 45 minutes, shaking sheet halfway through. Lightly coat small skillet with cooking spray and heat over medium. In small bowl beat 3 eggs, and scramble in skillet. Top roasted potatoes with scrambled eggs and ¼ sliced avocado. Enjoy with 1 cup whole milk.

Snack COTTAGE CHEESE PROTEIN BOWL

Top 1½ cups plain cottage cheese with 2 cups cubed pineapple and 2 Tbsp ground flaxseed.

Lunch Leftover HEARTY BEEF AND BEAN CHILI

Snack CHEESE, CRACKERS, FRUIT, AND NUTS

Eat 1 oz cheese of your choice, 6 whole grain crackers, 1 apple, and 24 almonds.

Dinner MEDITERRANEAN GRAIN BOWL (Leftover)

Snack YOGURT PARFAIT

Combine ½ cup plain full-fat Greek yogurt, ¼ cup low-sugar granola, ¾ cup berries, ½ sliced banana in alternating layers in a small bowl. Drizzle 1 Tbsp honey on top.

NUTRITION (PER DAY): 3,801 CALORIES | 241 G PROTEIN
360 G CARBOHYDRATES (69 G FIBER) | 164 G FAT

BEST MEALS FOR MUSCLE | WEEK 1

DAY 4

Breakfast BAGEL AND YOGURT
Toast 1 whole wheat bagel and top with 1½ Tbsp natural peanut butter and 1 sliced banana. Eat with 1 5.3-oz serving plain full-fat Greek yogurt.

Snack LOADED ENGLISH MUFFIN
Toast 1 whole wheat English muffin and fill with 2 Tbsp natural almond butter, 2 Tbsp dried cranberries, and 1 Tbsp unsweetened coconut flakes.

Lunch TURKEY WRAP
On 1 whole wheat 8-in. tortilla, layer ¼ sliced medium avocado, 6 oz low-sodium deli-sliced turkey, 1 slice Swiss cheese, and ½ sliced bell pepper. Fold in sides and roll up. Enjoy with 1 small orange.

Snack TRAIL MIX
Combine ¼ cup low-sugar granola with 6 cashews, 6 almonds, 4 walnut halves, and 1 Tbsp dark chocolate chips.

Dinner STEAK AND POTATOES
Preheat oven to 425°F. In large roasting pan, roast 1½ cups diced potatoes for 1 hour, turning occasionally until golden and fork-tender. Season 5 oz sirloin steak with 1 tsp each of basil, thyme, rosemary, and minced garlic. In skillet over medium high, add 1 Tbsp olive oil. Sear steak in skillet until desired doneness. Enjoy with 2 cups cooked green beans.

Snack BENTO BOX
Eat 1 oz cheese of your choice, 6 whole grain crackers, 16 grapes, and 24 almonds.

NUTRITION (PER DAY): 3,092 CALORIES | 171 G PROTEIN
329 G CARBOHYDRATES (56 G FIBER) | 134 G FAT

DAY 5

Breakfast BEAR-SIZED PB&J (p. 62)

Snack COTTAGE CHEESE PROTEIN BOWL
Top 1½ cups plain cottage cheese with 2 cups cubed pineapple and 2 Tbsp ground flaxseed.

Lunch TRIPLE DECKER CHICKEN CLUB (p. 66)

Snack CHEESE, CRACKERS, FRUIT, AND NUTS
Eat 1 oz cheese of your choice, 6 whole grain crackers, 1 apple, and 24 almonds.

Dinner SALMON ARUGULA SALAD (p.68)
Refrigerate remaining for Day 7 dinner.

Snack BANANA, PB, AND PRETZELS
Eat 1 sliced banana topped with 2 Tbsp natural peanut butter, and 13 pretzels.

NUTRITION (PER DAY): 3,307 CALORIES | 182 G PROTEIN
294 G CARBOHYDRATES (47 G FIBER) | 165 G FAT

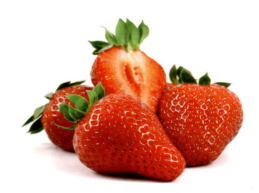

DAY 6

Breakfast
PROTEIN WAFFLE BREAKFAST SANDWICH

Toast 2 frozen protein waffles, such as Kodiak. Top with 2 scrambled eggs, 2 slices cooked turkey bacon, and 1 slice Cheddar cheese. Enjoy with 1 cup sliced strawberries.

Snack **LOADED ENGLISH MUFFIN**

Toast 1 whole wheat English muffin and fill with 2 Tbsp natural almond butter, 2 Tbsp dried cranberries, and 1 Tbsp unsweetened coconut flakes.

Lunch **TURKEY SANDWICH**

Toast 2 slices whole wheat bread and fill with 1 Tbsp sliced avocado, 6 oz low-sodium deli-sliced turkey, 1 slice Swiss cheese, a handful of spinach, and 1-2 slices each of onion and tomato. Eat with 1 small orange, 13 pretzels, and 1 cup whole milk.

Snack **TRAIL MIX**

Combine ¼ cup low-sugar granola with 6 cashews, 6 almonds, 4 walnut halves, and 1 Tbsp dark chocolate chips.

Dinner **VEGETARIAN STIR-FRY** (p. 81)

Snack **APPLE AND ALMOND BUTTER**

Slice 1 apple and dip in 2 Tbsp natural almond butter. Enjoy with 1 cup whole milk.

NUTRITION (PER DAY): 3,729 CALORIES | 181 G PROTEIN
390 G CARBOHYDRATES (37 G FIBER) | 174 G FAT

DAY 7

Breakfast **SWEET POTATO HASH BOWL**

Preheat oven to 425°F. On rimmed baking sheet, toss 1 cup diced sweet potatoes with 1 tsp olive oil, salt, and pepper. Bake until potatoes are crispy and fork-tender, about 45 minutes, shaking sheet halfway through. Lightly coat small skillet with cooking spray, and heat over medium. In small bowl beat 3 eggs, and scramble in skillet. Top roasted potatoes with scrambled eggs and ¼ sliced avocado. Enjoy with 1 cup whole milk.

Snack **COTTAGE CHEESE PROTEIN BOWL**

Top 1½ cups plain cottage cheese with 2 cups cubed pineapple and 2 Tbsp ground flaxseed.

Lunch **TURKEY SANDWICH**

Toast 2 slices whole wheat bread and fill with 1 Tbsp sliced avocado, 6 oz low-sodium deli-sliced turkey, 1 slice Swiss cheese, a handful of spinach, and 1-2 slices each of onion and tomato. Eat with 1 small orange, 13 pretzels, and 1 cup whole milk.

Snack **CHEESE, CRACKERS, FRUIT, AND NUTS**

Eat 1 oz cheese of your choice, 6 whole grain crackers, 1 apple, and 24 almonds.

Dinner **SALMON ARUGULA SALAD** (Leftover)

Snack **YOGURT PARFAIT**

Combine ½ cup plain full-fat Greek yogurt, ¼ cup low-sugar granola, ¾ cup berries, ½ sliced banana in alternating layers in a small bowl. Drizzle 1 Tbsp honey on top.

NUTRITION (PER DAY): 3,339 CALORIES | 189 G PROTEIN
313 G CARBOHYDRATES (58 G FIBER) | 158 G FAT

MH BEST MEALS FOR MUSCLE | WEEK 2

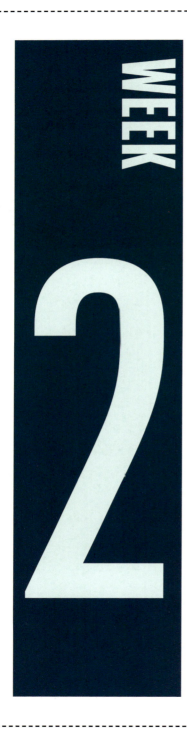

Shopping List

Check for leftover ingredients from Week 1 before purchasing new ingredients from the shopping list.

MEATS & PROTEINS

- 2 lbs **CHICKEN BREAST**
- 1 dozen **EGGS**
- 1 (10-oz) container **HUMMUS**
- 2 bone-in **PORK CHOPS**
- 3 (5-oz) fillets **SALMON**
- 10 oz **SHRIMP**
- 12 oz **LEAN STEAK**
- 1 (12-oz) package **TURKEY BACON**
- ½ lb low-sodium **TURKEY DELI MEAT**
- 1 box high-protein **FROZEN WAFFLES**, such as Kodiak

DAIRY

- ½ lb **CHEESE** of your choice
- 3 (16-oz) containers **COTTAGE CHEESE**
- 1 (8-oz) bag **SHREDDED PART-SKIM MOZZARELLA CHEESE**
- ¼ lb **SLICED CHEESE** of your choice
- 1 (8-oz) jar **MAYO**
- 1 pint **SKIM MILK**
- ½ gallon **WHOLE MILK**
- 1 (32-oz) container plus 2 (5.3-oz) containers **PLAIN FULL-FAT GREEK YOGURT**

PRODUCE

- 5 **APPLES**
- 1 (5-oz) container **ARUGULA**
- 2 bunches **ASPARAGUS**
- 2 medium **AVOCADOS**
- 4 **BANANAS**
- About ½ lb **BERRIES** of your choice
- 2 (6-oz) containers **BLACKBERRIES**
- 1 small **RED CABBAGE**
- 1 bunch **CHIVES**
- 1 (10-oz) bag **FROZEN CORN**
- 1 cup **GRAPES**
- 1 **LEMON**
- 1 small head **LETTUCE**
- 1 **LIME**
- 1 **ONION**
- 1 **RED ONION**
- 1 **RED PEPPER**
- 2 **PINEAPPLES**
- 1 (½-lb) bag **BABY POTATOES**
- 4-5 **SWEET POTATOES**
- 3 (8-oz) containers **RASPBERRIES**
- 1 (5-oz) container **SPINACH**
- 1 lb **STRAWBERRIES**
- 4 **TOMATOES**
- 2 (14.4-oz) bags **FROZEN STIR-FRY VEGETABLES**

PANTRY

1 (6.3-oz) bag **ALMONDS**
1 (16-oz) jar natural **ALMOND BUTTER**
1 (15-oz) can **BLACK BEANS**
2 (1-oz) packages **CASHEWS**
1 small jar **ANCHO CHILI POWDER**
1 (12-oz) bag **DARK CHOCOLATE CHIPS**
1 small jar **GROUND CINNAMON**
1 (8-oz) container **COCOA POWDER**
1 (12-oz) bag **UNSWEETENED COCONUT FLAKES**
1 (6-oz) package **DRIED CRANBERRIES**
1 small jar **CURRY POWDER**
1 (16-oz) package **GROUND FLAXSEED**
1 (12-oz) jar **HONEY**
1 (12-oz) package **HIGH-PROTEIN GRANOLA**
1 (12-oz) package **LOW-SUGAR GRANOLA**
1 small jar **PURE MAPLE SYRUP**
1 (18-oz) container **QUICK-COOKING OATS**
1 small bottle **OLIVE OIL**
1 (16-oz) jar **NATURAL PEANUT BUTTER**
1 (6-oz) jar prepared **PESTO**
1 (12-oz) box **RAISINS**
1 small jar **RED PEPPER FLAKES**
1 (2-lb) bag **BROWN RICE**
SALT and **PEPPER**
1 (15.5-oz) jar **SALSA**
1 (16-oz) jar **MANGO SALSA**
1 small bottle **TERIYAKI SAUCE**
1 package **CORN TORTILLAS**
1 small bottle **BALSAMIC VINEGAR**
1 (12-oz) bottle **RED WINE VINEGAR**
3 oz **WALNUT HALVES**
1 (8.5-oz) box **WHOLE GRAIN CRACKERS**, such as Triscuits
1 **WHOLE WHEAT BAGEL**
1 (5-oz) bag **WHOLE WHEAT CROUTONS**
4 **WHOLE WHEAT ENGLISH MUFFINS**
1 package **WHOLE WHEAT PITAS**
1 package **WHOLE WHEAT 8-IN. TORTILLAS**

MEAL PREP

Store all items in air-tight containers. If perishable, keep in your refrigerator.

ON DAY 7

Cook 6 oz chicken breast.
Prep 3 servings of Trail Mix (p.50).
Slice 1 cup strawberries.
Cube 2 cups pineapple.

ON DAY 10

Dice 2½ cups sweet potatoes.
Cook 14 oz chicken breast.
Cube 2 cups pineapple.

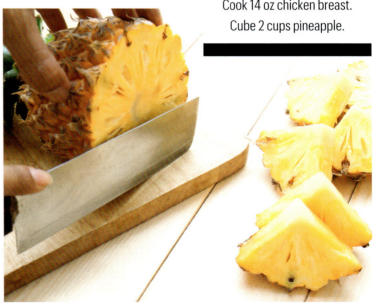

BEST MEALS FOR MUSCLE | WEEK 2

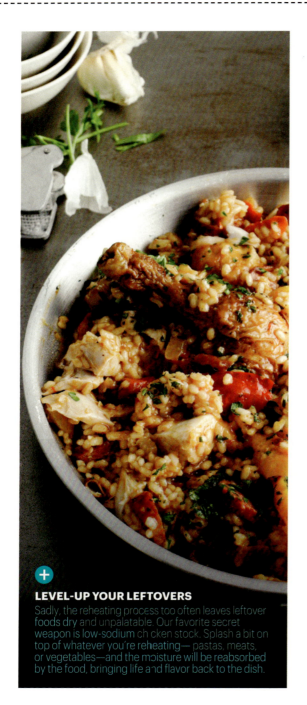

LEVEL-UP YOUR LEFTOVERS
Sadly, the reheating process too often leaves leftover foods dry and unpalatable. Our favorite secret weapon is low-sodium chicken stock. Splash a bit on top of whatever you're reheating— pastas, meats, or vegetables—and the moisture will be reabsorbed by the food, bringing life and flavor back to the dish.

DAY 8

Breakfast PROTEIN OATMEAL

Cook 1 cup quick-cooking oats according to package directions. Place in small bowl and stir in 1 cup plain full-fat Greek yogurt, 1 tsp honey, 8 chopped walnut halves, and ¾ cup blackberries.

Snack YOGURT PARFAIT

Combine ¾ cup plain full-fat Greek yogurt, ¼ cup low-sugar granola, ¾ cup raspberries, ½ sliced banana in alternating layers in a small bowl. Drizzle 1 Tbsp honey on top.

Lunch CHICKEN AVOCADO SALAD

In large bowl, toss together 2 cups spinach, 6 oz cooked chicken breast, 2 Tbsp avocado, ¼ cup shredded part-skim mozzarella cheese, ½ cup whole wheat croutons, and 4 Tbsp balsamic vinaigrette.

Snack TRAIL MIX

Combine ¼ cup low-sugar granola with 6 cashews, 6 almonds, 4 walnut halves, and 1 Tbsp dark chocolate chips.

Dinner STEAK BURRITOS

In medium skillet, sear 12 oz lean steak until desired doneness. Let rest and dice. Cook ⅔ cup brown rice according to package directions. Prep additional fillings: 1 cup black beans, rinsed and drained, ½ cup diced tomato, ½ cup corn, 4 Tbsp avocado, and 4 Tbsp salsa. Divide half filling between 2 whole wheat 8-in. tortillas. Fold in sides and roll up. Makes 2 servings. Refrigerate leftovers for Day 9 lunch.

Snack LOADED ENGLISH MUFFIN

Toast 1 whole wheat English muffin and fill with 2 Tbsp natural almond butter, 2 Tbsp dried cranberries, and 1 Tbsp unsweetened coconut flakes.

NUTRITION (PER DAY): 3,460 CALORIES | 213 G PROTEIN
331 G CARBOHYDRATES (63 G FIBER) | 151 G FAT

DAY 9

Breakfast PROTEIN WAFFLE BREAKFAST SANDWICH

Toast 2 frozen protein waffles, such as Kodiak. Top with 2 scrambled eggs, 2 slices cooked turkey bacon, and 1 slice Cheddar cheese. Enjoy with 1 cup sliced strawberries.

Snack CHEESE, CRACKERS, FRUIT, AND NUTS

Eat 1 oz cheese of your choice, 6 whole grain crackers, 1 apple, and 24 almonds.

Lunch STEAK BURRITOS (Leftover)

Snack COTTAGE CHEESE PROTEIN BOWL

Top 1½ cups plain cottage cheese with 2 cups cubed pineapple and 2 Tbsp ground flaxseed.

Dinner CHICKEN MOLE TACOS (p. 70)

Serve with ½ sliced avocado.

Snack APPLE AND ALMOND BUTTER

Slice 1 apple and dip in 2 Tbsp natural almond butter. Enjoy with 1 cup whole milk.

NUTRITION (PER DAY): 3,490 CALORIES | 211 G PROTEIN
317 G CARBOHYDRATES (60 G FIBER) | 164 G FAT

DAY 10

Breakfast STRENGTH STACK

In medium bowl, mix 1 banana, 1 egg and 2 egg whites, ¼ cup quick-cooking oats, and ¼ cup cottage cheese. Lightly coat small skillet with cooking spray and heat over medium. Add half the batter and cook about 3 minutes, or until bubbles form. Flip and cook 3 minutes. Transfer to plate and repeat with remaining batter. Top with ¾ cup berries and 2 Tbsp maple syrup. Enjoy with 1 cup whole milk.

Snack YOGURT PARFAIT

Combine ¾ cup plain full-fat Greek yogurt, ¼ cup low-sugar granola, ¾ cup raspberries, ½ sliced banana in alternating layers in a small bowl. Drizzle 1 Tbsp honey on top.

Lunch CHICKEN MOLE TACOS (Leftover)

Serve with ½ sliced avocado.

Snack TRAIL MIX

Combine ¼ cup low-sugar granola with 6 cashews, 6 almonds, 4 walnut halves, and 1 Tbsp dark chocolate chips.

Dinner MUSTARD MAPLE PORK CHOPS (p. 72)

Cook 2 sweet potatoes and 1 bunch asparagus. Eat half with 1 pork chop. Refrigerate remaining for Day 12 lunch.

Snack BENTO BOX

Eat 1 oz cheese of your choice, 6 whole grain crackers, 16 grapes, and 24 almonds.

NUTRITION (PER DAY): 2,768 CALORIES | 160 G PROTEIN
315 G CARBOHYDRATES (42 G FIBER) | 105 G FAT

BEST MEALS FOR MUSCLE | WEEK 2

DAY 11

Breakfast SWEET POTATO HASH BOWL

Preheat oven to 425°F. On rimmed baking sheet, toss 1 cup diced sweet potatoes with 1 tsp olive oil, salt, and pepper. Bake until potatoes are crispy and fork-tender, about 45 minutes, shaking sheet halfway through. Lightly coat small skillet with cooking spray, and heat over medium. In small bowl beat 3 eggs, and scramble in skillet. Top roasted potatoes with scrambled eggs and ¼ sliced avocado. Enjoy with 1 cup whole milk.

Snack CHEESE, CRACKERS, FRUIT, AND NUTS

Eat 1 oz cheese of your choice, 6 whole grain crackers, 1 apple, and 24 almonds.

Lunch CURRIED CHICKEN SALAD PITA

In medium bowl, mix 8 oz cooked and shredded chicken breast, 4 Tbsp mayo, ¼ cup raisins, 2 tsp curry powder, and 2 Tbsp minced chives. Spoon half into ½ whole wheat pita. Refrigerate remaining for Day 13 lunch.

Snack COTTAGE CHEESE PROTEIN BOWL

Top 1½ cups plain cottage cheese with 2 cups cubed pineapple and 2 Tbsp ground flaxseed.

Dinner MANGO SALMON

Cook 5 oz salmon. Top with 3 Tbsp mango salsa. Enjoy with 1½ cups cubed cooked sweet potatoes and 12 cooked asparagus spears.

Snack MINI SANDWICH

Toast 1 whole wheat English muffin and fill with 4 oz low-sodium turkey deli meat, 1 slice cheese, 2 Tbsp avocado, 2 Tbsp hummus, lettuce, onion, and tomato.

NUTRITION (PER DAY): 3,328 CALORIES | 208 G PROTEIN
314 G CARBOHYDRATES (51 G FIBER) | 146 G FAT

DAY 12

Breakfast BEAR-SIZED PB&J (p.62)

Snack YOGURT PARFAIT

Combine ¾ cup plain full-fat Greek yogurt, ¼ cup low-sugar granola, ¾ cup raspberries, ½ sliced banana in alternating layers in a small bowl. Drizzle 1 Tbsp honey on top.

Lunch MUSTARD MAPLE PORK CHOPS (Leftover)

Serve with leftover sweet potatoes and asparagus.

Snack TRAIL MIX

Combine ¼ cup low-sugar granola with 6 cashews, 6 almonds, 4 walnut halves, and 1 Tbsp dark chocolate chips.

Dinner SHRIMP TERIYAKI BOWL

Cook 10 oz shrimp with 4 cups frozen stir-fry vegetables, and make 2 cups brown rice according to package directions. Plate ½ the rice and top with ½ the vegetables, 5 oz shrimp, and 2 Tbsp low-sodium teriyaki sauce. Makes 2 servings. Refrigerate remaining for Day 13 dinner.

Snack LOADED ENGLISH MUFFIN

Toast 1 whole wheat English muffin and fill with 2 Tbsp natural almond butter, 2 Tbsp dried cranberries, and 1 Tbsp unsweetened coconut flakes.

NUTRITION (PER DAY): 3,014 CALORIES | 164 G PROTEIN
337 G CARBOHYDRATES (61 G FIBER) | 119 G FAT

DAY 13

Breakfast PROTEIN OATMEAL
Cook 1 cup quick-cooking oats according to package directions. Place in small bowl and stir in 1 cup plain full-fat Greek yogurt, 1 tsp honey, 8 chopped walnut halves, and ¾ cup blackberries.

Snack CHEESE, CRACKERS, FRUIT, AND NUTS
Eat 1 oz cheese of your choice, 6 whole grain crackers, 1 apple, and 24 almonds.

Lunch CURRIED CHICKEN SALAD PITA (Leftover)

Snack COTTAGE CHEESE PROTEIN BOWL
Top 1½ cups plain cottage cheese with 2 cups cubed pineapple and 2 Tbsp ground flaxseed.

Dinner SHRIMP TERIYAKI BOWL (Leftover)

Snack APPLE AND ALMOND BUTTER
Slice 1 apple and dip in 2 Tbsp natural almond butter. Enjoy with 1 cup whole milk.

NUTRITION (PER DAY): 3,579 CALORIES | 205 G PROTEIN | 374 G CARBOHYDRATES (67 G FIBER) | 152 G FAT

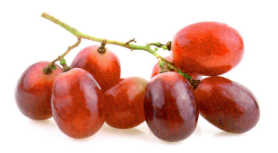

DAY 14

Breakfast BAGEL AND YOGURT
Toast 1 whole wheat bagel and top with 1½ Tbsp natural peanut butter and 1 sliced banana. Eat with 1 5.3-oz serving plain full-fat Greek yogurt.

Snack BENTO BOX
Eat 1 oz cheese of your choice, 6 whole grain crackers, 16 grapes, and 24 almonds.

Lunch CHICKEN AVOCADO SALAD WRAP
On 1 whole wheat 8-in. tortilla, layer 2 cups spinach, 6 oz cooked chicken breast, 2 Tbsp sliced avocado, ¼ cup shredded part-skim mozzarella cheese. Drizzle 4 Tbsp balsamic vinaigrette on top. Fold in sides and roll up.

Snack TRAIL MIX
Combine ¼ cup low-sugar granola with 6 cashews, 6 almonds, 4 walnut halves, and 1 Tbsp dark chocolate chips.

Dinner SALMON ARUGULA SALAD (p.68)

Snack MINI SANDWICH
Toast 1 whole wheat English muffin and fill with 4 oz low-sodium turkey deli meat, 1 slice cheese, 2 Tbsp avocado, 2 Tbsp hummus, lettuce, onion, and tomato.

NUTRITION (PER DAY): 3,273 CALORIES | 215 G PROTEIN | 271 G CARBOHYDRATES (49 G FIBER) | 157 G FAT

BEST MEALS FOR MUSCLE | WEEK 3

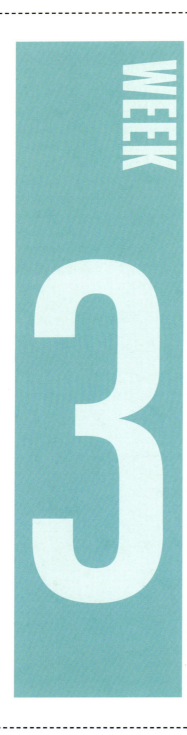

Shopping List

Check for leftover ingredients from Week 2 before purchasing new ingredients from the shopping list.

MEATS & PROTEINS

- 1 (12-oz) package **THICK BACON**
- 2 (6-oz) 96% **LEAN GROUND BEEF PATTIES**
- 3 (6-oz) **CHICKEN BREASTS**
- 6 oz **CHICKEN SAUSAGE**
- ½ dozen **EGGS**
- 1 (16-oz) container **LIQUID EGG WHITES**
- 1 (10-oz) container **HUMMUS**
- 4 (6-oz) pieces **SALMON**
- 2 small **TILAPIA FILLETS**
- 1 (12-oz) package **TURKEY BACON**
- ¼ lb low-sodium **TURKEY DELI MEAT**
- 1 box high-protein **FROZEN WAFFLES**, such as Kodiak

DAIRY

- 2 oz **CHEESE** of your choice
- 3 (16-oz) containers **PLAIN COTTAGE CHEESE**
- ¼ lb **PROVOLONE CHEESE**
- ¼ lb **SLICED CHEESE** of your choice
- ¼ lb **SWISS CHEESE**
- 1 (8-oz) jar **MAYO**
- 1 pint **SKIM MILK**
- ¼ gallon **WHOLE MILK**
- 1 (32-oz) container **PLAIN FULL-FAT GREEK YOGURT**

PRODUCE

- 4 **APPLES**
- 4 **AVOCADOS**
- 6 **BANANAS**
- About 1 lb **BERRIES** of your choice
- 2 (6-oz) containers **BLACKBERRIES**
- 1 lb **BROCCOLI RABE**
- 1 large **CAULIFLOWER HEAD**
- 1 small bunch **CELERY**
- 1 head **GARLIC**
- 1 (2-in.) piece **FRESH GINGER**
- 1 **GRAPEFRUIT**
- 1 cup **GRAPES**
- 1 **JALAPEÑO**
- 1 head **LETTUCE**
- 1 **LIME**
- 1 (8-oz) container **MUSHROOMS**
- 2 **ONIONS**
- 1 small **RED ONION**
- 2 **ORANGES**
- 1 small bunch **PARSLEY**
- 1 **BELL PEPPER**
- 2 **PINEAPPLES**
- 3 large **SWEET POTATOES**
- 2 (6-oz) containers **RASPBERRIES**
- 1 small bunch **SCALLIONS**
- 1 (16-oz) container spinach, plus 1 (5-oz) container **SPINACH**
- 2 **TOMATOES**

PANTRY

1 (6.3-oz) bag **ALMONDS**

1 (16-oz) jar natural **ALMOND BUTTER**

1 (1-oz) package **CASHEWS**

1 (2.5-oz) jar **CAPERS**

1 (12-oz) bag **DARK CHOCOLATE CHIPS**

1 small loaf **CIABATTA BREAD**

1 (12-oz) bag **UNSWEETENED COCONUT FLAKES**

1 bottle **COOKING SPRAY**

1 (6-oz) package **DRIED CRANBERRIES**

1 small jar **GROUND CUMIN**

1 (16-oz) package **GROUND FLAXSEED**

1 (12-oz) package **HIGH-PROTEIN GRANOLA**

1 (12-oz) package **LOW-SUGAR GRANOLA**

1 (12-oz) jar **HONEY**

1 container **HOT SAUCE** or **SALSA**

1 small jar pickled **JALAPEÑOS**

1 small container **KETCHUP**

1 (18-oz) container **QUICK-COOKING OATS**

1 bottle **CANOLA OIL**

1 small bottle **OLIVE OIL**

1 box **PASTA**

1 (16-oz) jar **NATURAL PEANUT BUTTER**

1 package **PITA**

1 (16-oz) bag **PRETZELS**

1 (1-lb) package **WHITE RICE**

SALT and **PEPPER**

1 (3-oz) bag **DRY-PACKED SUN-DRIED TOMATOES**

1 package **WHOLE WHEAT TORTILLAS**

2 cans **TUNA PACKED IN WATER**

1.5 oz **WALNUT HALVES**

1 (8.5-oz) box **WHOLE GRAIN CRACKERS**, such as Triscuits

2 **WHOLE WHEAT BAGELS**

1 package **WHOLE WHEAT BURGER BUNS**

1 package **WHOLE WHEAT ENGLISH MUFFINS**

MEAL PREP

Store all items in air-tight containers. If perishable, keep in your refrigerator.

ON DAY 14

Cook 6 oz chicken breast.

Cube 4 cups pineapple.

Prep 2 servings Trail Mix (p. 56).

ON DAY 17

Dice 1 cup sweet potatoes.

Dice 2 stalks celery, and divide into separate containers.

Cube 4 cups pineapple.

Cook 6 oz chicken breast.

BEST MEALS FOR MUSCLE | WEEK 3

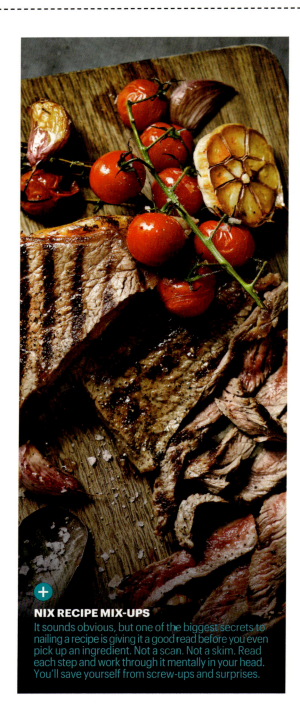

NIX RECIPE MIX-UPS
It sounds obvious, but one of the biggest secrets to nailing a recipe is giving it a good read before you even pick up an ingredient. Not a scan. Not a skim. Read each step and work through it mentally in your head. You'll save yourself from screw-ups and surprises.

DAY 15

Breakfast VEGGIE OMELET AND BAGEL
Heat large skillet coated with cooking spray over medium low. Sauté ⅓ cup each spinach, sliced mushrooms, and diced onion until tender. Transfer to bowl. Coat skillet with additional cooking spray, if needed. Add 1 cup liquid egg whites and cooked vegetables to skillet. Cook until set. Top with hot sauce or salsa. Enjoy with 1 cup whole milk and 1 whole wheat bagel topped with 1 Tbsp natural peanut butter and ½ sliced banana.

Snack BANANA, PB, AND PRETZELS
Eat 1 sliced banana topped with 2 Tbsp natural peanut butter, and 13 pretzels.

Lunch CHICKEN PROVOLONE SANDWICH
Toast 2 slices ciabatta bread. Spread 1 Tbsp mayo on one slice and 4 Tbsp mashed avocado on the other. Fill with 6 oz cooked chicken breast, 1 slice provolone cheese, spinach, onion, and tomato.

Snack COTTAGE CHEESE PROTEIN BOWL
Top 1½ cups plain cottage cheese with 2 cups cubed pineapple and 2 Tbsp ground flaxseed.

Dinner LIME TILAPIA WITH CITRUS-AVOCADO SALSA (p.74)
Refrigerate remaining for Day 16 lunch.

Snack TRAIL MIX
Combine ¼ cup low-sugar granola with 6 cashews, 6 almonds, 4 walnut halves, and 1 Tbsp dark chocolate chips.

NUTRITION (PER DAY): 3,237 CALORIES | 224 G PROTEIN | 26 G CARBOHYDRATES (37 G FIBER) | 123 G FAT

DAY 16

Breakfast BEAR-SIZED PB&J (p. 62)

Snack APPLE AND ALMOND BUTTER
Slice 1 apple and dip in 2 Tbsp natural almond butter. Enjoy with 1 cup whole milk.

Lunch LIME TILAPIA WITH CITRUS-AVOCADO SALSA (Leftover)

Snack LOADED ENGLISH MUFFIN
Toast 1 whole wheat English muffin and fill with 2 Tbsp natural almond butter, 2 Tbsp dried cranberries, and 1 Tbsp unsweetened coconut flakes.

Dinner BLT BURGER
Heat medium skillet coated with cooking spray over medium. Cook 1 6-oz 96 percent lean ground beef patty until desired doneness. Toast 1 whole wheat burger bun. Top bun with burger, 1 slice Swiss cheese, 2 slices cooked turkey bacon, 2 Tbsp avocado, 2 Tbsp ketchup, 1 Tbsp mushrooms, lettuce, onion, and tomato.

Snack YOGURT PARFAIT
Combine ¾ cup plain full-fat Greek yogurt, ¼ cup low-sugar granola, ¾ cup raspberries, ½ sliced banana in alternating layers in a small bowl. Drizzle 1 Tbsp honey on top.

NUTRITION (PER DAY): 2,664 CALORIES | 163 G PROTEIN
253 G CARBOHYDRATES (39 G FIBER) | 121 G FAT

DAY 17

Breakfast PROTEIN OATMEAL
Cook 1 cup quick-cooking oats according to package directions. Place in small bowl and stir in 1 cup plain full-fat Greek yogurt, 1 tsp honey, 8 chopped walnut halves, and ¾ cup blackberries.

Snack BANANA, PB, AND PRETZELS
Eat 1 sliced banana topped with 2 Tbsp natural peanut butter, and 13 pretzels.

Lunch ORANGE SWEET POTATO SALAD WITH CHICKEN (p. 80)
Refrigerate remaining for Day 19 lunch.

Snack COTTAGE CHEESE PROTEIN BOWL
Top 1½ cups plain cottage cheese with 2 cups cubed pineapple and 2 Tbsp ground flaxseed.

Dinner SEARED SALMON WITH ROASTED CAULIFLOWER (p. 76)
Refrigerate remaining for Day 19 dinner.

Snack BENTO BOX
Eat 1 oz cheese of your choice, 6 whole grain crackers, 16 grapes, and 24 almonds.

NUTRITION (PER DAY): 3,386 CALORIES | 198 G PROTEIN
318 G CARBOHYDRATES (56 G FIBER) | 160 FAT

BEST MEALS FOR MUSCLE | WEEK 3

DAY 18

Breakfast SWEET POTATO HASH BOWL

Preheat oven to 425°F. On rimmed baking sheet, toss 1 cup diced sweet potatoes with 1 tsp olive oil, salt, and pepper. Bake until potatoes are crispy and fork-tender, about 45 minutes, shaking sheet halfway through. Lightly coat small skillet with cooking spray, and heat over medium. In small bowl beat 3 eggs, and scramble in skillet. Top roasted potatoes with scrambled eggs and ¼ sliced avocado. Enjoy with 1 cup whole milk.

Snack APPLE AND ALMOND BUTTER

Slice 1 apple and dip in 2 Tbsp natural almond butter. Enjoy with 1 cup whole milk.

Lunch TUNA SALAD PITA

In small bowl, combine 1 stalk diced celery, 1½ Tbsp mayo, 1 Tbsp pickled jalapeño, and ¼ tsp salt and pepper. Mix in 1 can drained tuna packed in water. Spoon into ½ whole wheat pita and top with ½ sliced avocado.

Snack LOADED ENGLISH MUFFIN

Toast 1 whole wheat English muffin and fill with 2 Tbsp natural almond butter, 2 Tbsp dried cranberries, and 1 Tbsp unsweetened coconut flakes.

Dinner BLT BURGER

Heat medium skillet coated with cooking spray over medium. Cook 1 6-oz 96 percent lean ground beef patty until desired doneness. Toast 1 whole wheat burger bun. Top bun with burger, 1 slice Swiss cheese, 2 slices cooked turkey bacon, 2 Tbsp avocado, 2 Tbsp ketchup, 1 Tbsp mushrooms, lettuce, onion, and tomato.

Snack YOGURT PARFAIT

Combine ¾ cup plain full-fat Greek yogurt, ¼ cup low-sugar granola, ¾ cup raspberries, ½ sliced banana in alternating layers in a small bowl. Drizzle 1 Tbsp honey on top.

NUTRITION (PER DAY): 3,375 CALORIES | 193 G PROTEIN
283 G CARBOHYDRATES (50 G FIBER) | 172 G FAT

DAY 19

Breakfast VEGGIE OMELET AND BAGEL

Heat large skillet coated with cooking spray over medium low. Sauté ⅓ cup each spinach, sliced mushrooms, and diced onion until tender. Transfer to bowl. Coat skillet with additional cooking spray, if needed. Add 1 cup liquid egg whites and cooked vegetables to skillet. Cook until set. Enjoy with 1 cup skim milk and 1 whole wheat bagel topped with 1 Tbsp natural peanut butter and ½ sliced banana.

Snack BANANA, PB, AND PRETZELS

Eat 1 sliced banana topped with 2 Tbsp natural peanut butter, and 13 pretzels.

Lunch ORANGE SWEET POTATO SALAD WITH CHICKEN (Leftover)

Snack COTTAGE CHEESE PROTEIN BOWL

Top 1½ cups plain cottage cheese with 2 cups cubed pineapple and 2 Tbsp ground flaxseed.

Dinner SEARED SALMON WITH ROASTED CAULIFLOWER (Leftover)

Snack MINI SANDWICH

Toast 1 whole wheat English muffin and fill with 4 oz low-sodium turkey deli meat, 1 slice cheese of your choice, 2 Tbsp avocado, 2 Tbsp hummus, lettuce, onion, and tomato.

NUTRITION (PER DAY): 3,441 CALORIES
243 G PROTEIN | 331 G CARBOHYDRATES (57 G FIBER)
130 G FAT

DAY 20

Breakfast BEAR-SIZED PB&J (p. 62)

Snack APPLE AND ALMOND BUTTER
Slice 1 apple and dip in 2 Tbsp natural almond butter. Enjoy with 1 cup skim milk.

Lunch TUNA SALAD PITA
In small bowl, combine 1 stalk diced celery, 1½ Tbsp mayo, 1 Tbsp pickled jalapeño, and ¼ tsp salt and pepper. Mix in 1 can drained tuna packed in water. Spoon into ½ whole wheat pita and top with ½ sliced avocado.

Snack LOADED ENGLISH MUFFIN
Toast 1 whole wheat English muffin and fill with 2 Tbsp natural almond butter, 2 Tbsp dried cranberries, and 1 Tbsp unsweetened coconut flakes.

Dinner SAUSAGE AND BROCCOLI RABE PASTA (p. 78)
Refrigerate remaining for Day 21 dinner.

Snack BENTO BOX
Eat 1 oz cheese of your choice, 6 whole grain crackers, 16 grapes, and 24 almonds.

NUTRITION (PER DAY): 3,139 CALORIES | 149 G PROTEIN
278 G CARBOHYDRATES (53 G FIBER) | 172 G FAT

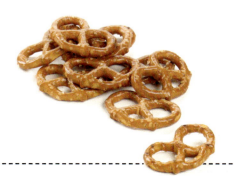

DAY 21

Breakfast PROTEIN OATMEAL
Cook 1 cup quick-cooking oats according to package directions. Place in small bowl and stir in 1 cup plain full-fat Greek yogurt, 1 tsp honey, 8 chopped walnut halves, and ¾ cup blackberries.

Snack BANANA, PB, AND PRETZELS
Eat 1 sliced banana topped with 2 Tbsp natural peanut butter, and 13 pretzels.

Lunch CHICKEN PROVOLONE WRAP
On 1 whole wheat 8-in tortilla, spread 1 Tbsp mayo and 4 Tbsp avocado. Top with 6 oz cooked and sliced chicken breast, 1 slice provolone cheese, spinach, onion, and tomato. Fold in sides and roll up.

Snack COTTAGE CHEESE PROTEIN BOWL
Top 1½ cups plain cottage cheese with 2 cups cubed pineapple and 2 Tbsp ground flaxseed.

Dinner SAUSAGE AND BROCCOLI RABE PASTA (Leftover)

Snack TRAIL MIX
Combine ¼ cup low-sugar granola with 6 cashews, 6 almonds, 4 walnut halves, and 1 Tbsp dark chocolate chips.

NUTRITION (PER DAY): 3,190 CALORIES | 192 G PROTEIN
311 G CARBOHYDRATES (48 G FIBER) | 139 G FAT

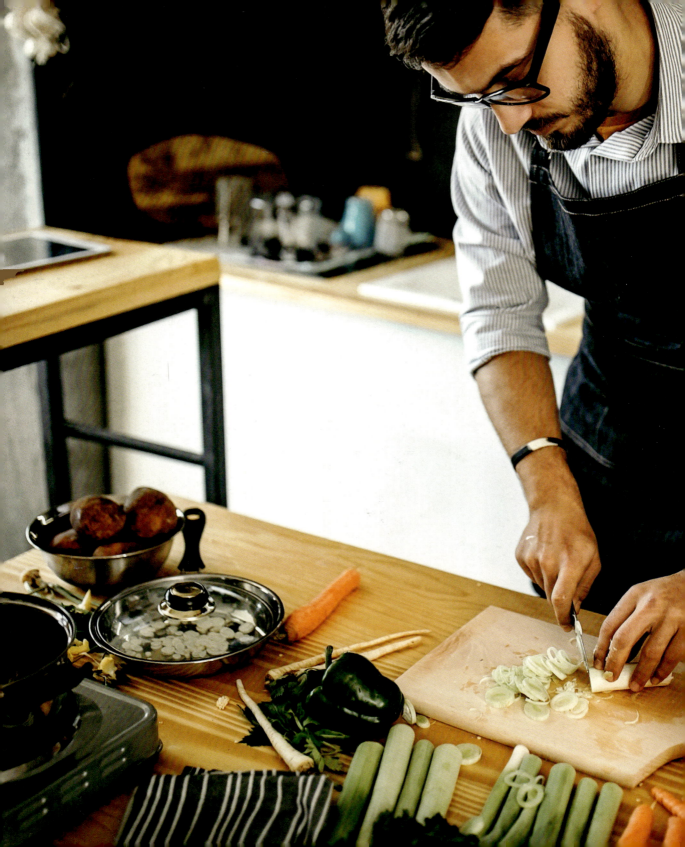

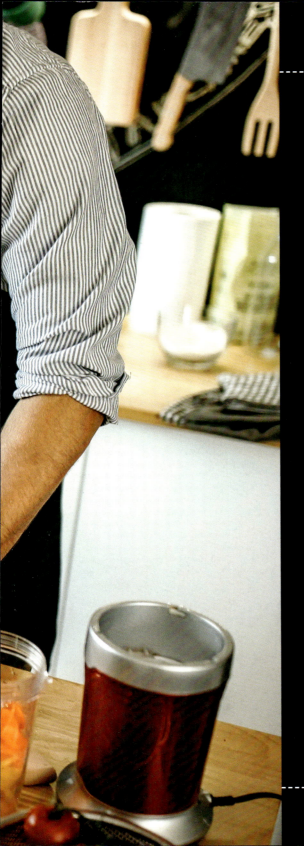

MEAL PLAN
Recipes

- **62** BEAR-SIZED PB&J
- **64** HEARTY BEEF AND BEAN CHILI
- **66** TRIPLE DECKER CHICKEN CLUB
- **68** SALMON ARUGULA SALAD
- **70** CHICKEN MOLE TACOS
- **72** MUSTARD MAPLE PORK CHOPS
- **74** LIME TILAPIA WITH CITRUS-AVOCADO SALSA
- **76** SEARED SALMON WITH ROASTED CAULIFLOWER
- **78** SAUSAGE AND BROCCOLI RABE PASTA
- **80** ORANGE SWEET POTATO SALAD WITH CHICKEN
- **81** VEGETARIAN STIR-FRY

MH BEST MEALS FOR MUSCLE

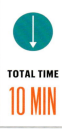

TOTAL TIME
10 MIN

BEAR-SIZED PB&J

WHAT YOU'LL NEED

- 2 HIGH-PROTEIN FREEZER WAFFLES (such as Kodiak)
- 2 TBSP NATURAL PEANUT BUTTER
- ⅓ CUP BERRIES, CHOPPED
- 2 TBSP HIGH-PROTEIN GRANOLA (such as Nature Valley)

HOW TO MAKE IT

▸ Toast waffles according to package directions. While they're warm, spread the peanut butter over one waffle. Top with berries, granola, and other waffle. Smush before eating.

MAKES 1 SANDWICH.

NUTRITION PER SERVING
682 CALORIES | 27 G PROTEIN | 54 G CARBS (10 G FIBER) | 41 G FAT

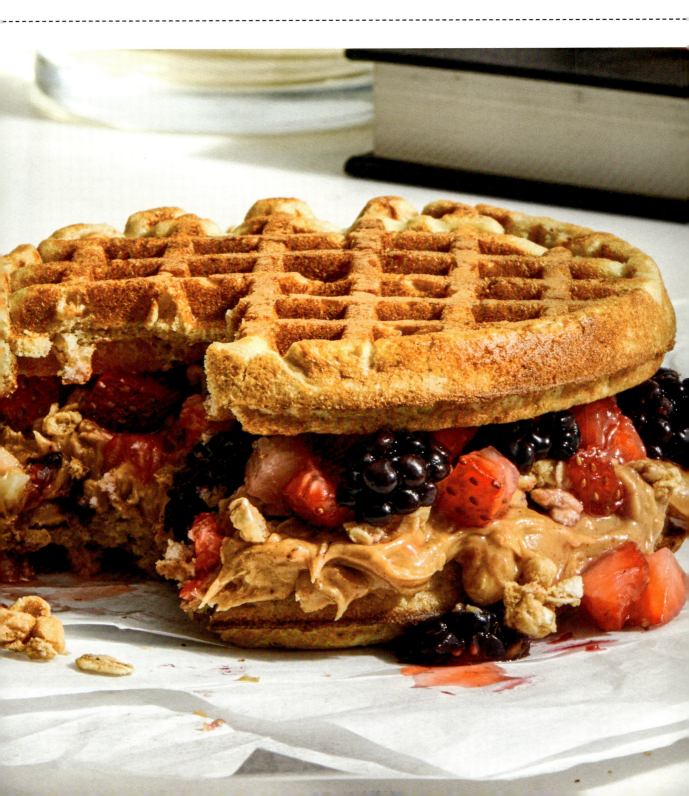

MH BEST MEALS FOR MUSCLE

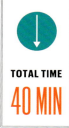

TOTAL TIME
40 MIN

HEARTY BEEF AND BEAN CHILI

WHAT YOU'LL NEED

- 1 TBSP OLIVE OIL, DIVIDED
- ½ LB LEAN GROUND BEEF
- 1 TSP GROUND CUMIN
- 1 TSP CHILI POWDER
- KOSHER SALT AND PEPPER TO TASTE
- ½ YELLOW ONION, FINELY CHOPPED
- 1 CLOVE GARLIC, PRESSED
- ½ LB TOMATOES, FINELY CHOPPED
- 1 15-OZ CAN CANNELLINI BEANS, RINSED
- ½ AVOCADO (for serving)

HOW TO MAKE IT

▶ Heat ½ Tbsp oil in large pot over medium. Add beef, cumin, chili powder, and ½ tsp each salt and pepper. Cook, breaking up beef, until browned, about 10 minutes. Transfer beef to plate.

▶ Return pot to medium heat; add remaining ½ Tbsp olive oil and onion, and cook until tender, 4 to 5 minutes. Stir in garlic and cook 1 minute. Add tomatoes and cook until they release their juices, about 5 minutes. Add 2 cups water and simmer until slightly thickened, about 10 minutes.

▶ Place half the beans in small bowl and mash with fork. Add them, the whole beans, and reserved beef to the pot and heat through.

MAKES 2 SERVINGS.

NUTRITION PER SERVING
629 CALORIES | 41 G PROTEIN | 59 G CARBOHYDRATES (16 G FIBER) | 27 G FAT

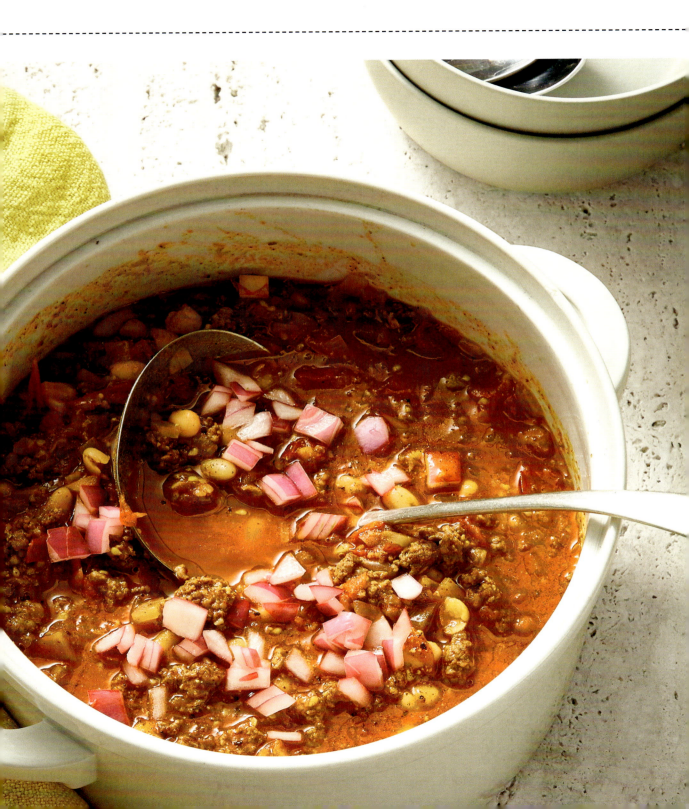

MH BEST MEALS FOR MUSCLE

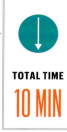

TOTAL TIME
10 MIN

TRIPLE DECKER CHICKEN CLUB

WHAT YOU'LL NEED

- 3 SLICES WHOLE WHEAT BREAD, TOASTED
- ½ TSP MUSTARD
- ½ TSP MAYO
- 1 SLICE CHEDDAR CHEESE
- 2 LETTUCE LEAVES
- 4 SLICES TOMATO
- 3 OZ ROTISSERIE CHICKEN

HOW TO MAKE IT

▶ Spread mustard on 2 toast slices and mayo on each side of 1 slice. Top 1 mustard-coated slice with Cheddar cheese, 1 lettuce leaf, 2 tomato slices, and 1 ½ oz rotisserie chicken. Top stack with the mayo-coated toast; then repeat with the same filling. Top with remaining toast.

▶ Cut diagonally down the middle.

MAKES 1 SERVING.

NUTRITION PER SERVING

508 CALORIES | 45 G PROTEIN | 38 G CARBOHYDRATES (6 G FIBER) | 19 G FAT

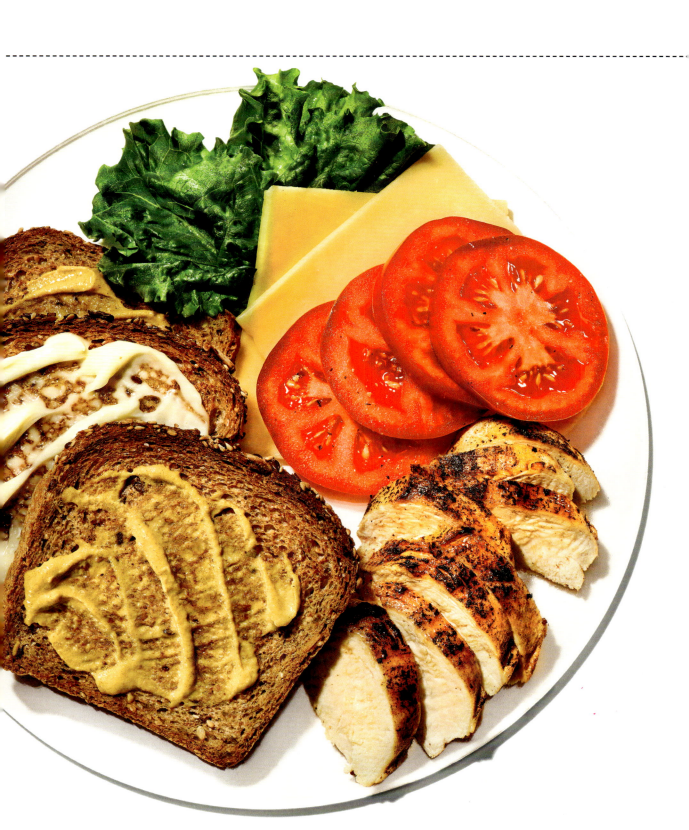

MH BEST MEALS FOR MUSCLE

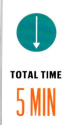

TOTAL TIME
5 MIN

SALMON ARUGULA SALAD

WHAT YOU'LL NEED

DRESSING
- 3 TBSP PREPARED PESTO
- 2 TBSP OLIVE OIL
- 2 TBSP RED WINE VINEGAR
- 2 TSP LEMON ZEST
- ¼ TSP RED PEPPER FLAKES

SALAD
- 4 CUPS ARUGULA LEAVES
- 2 TOMATOES, SLICED
- 2 5-OZ FILLETS GRILLED SALMON
- 2 OZ GOAT CHEESE
- 2 CUPS ROASTED BABY POTATOES

HOW TO MAKE IT

▶ Whisk all dressing ingredients in a small bowl until combined.

▶ In large bowl, toss all salad ingredients, except salmon, with dressing. (Note: If saving leftovers, only dress what you will eat immediately.) Divide in half and top each portion with 1 salmon fillet and 2 Tbsp pesto.

MAKES 2 SERVINGS.

NUTRITION PER SERVING
647 CALORIES | 42 G PROTEIN | 35 G CARBOHYDRATES (6 G FIBER) | 38 G FAT

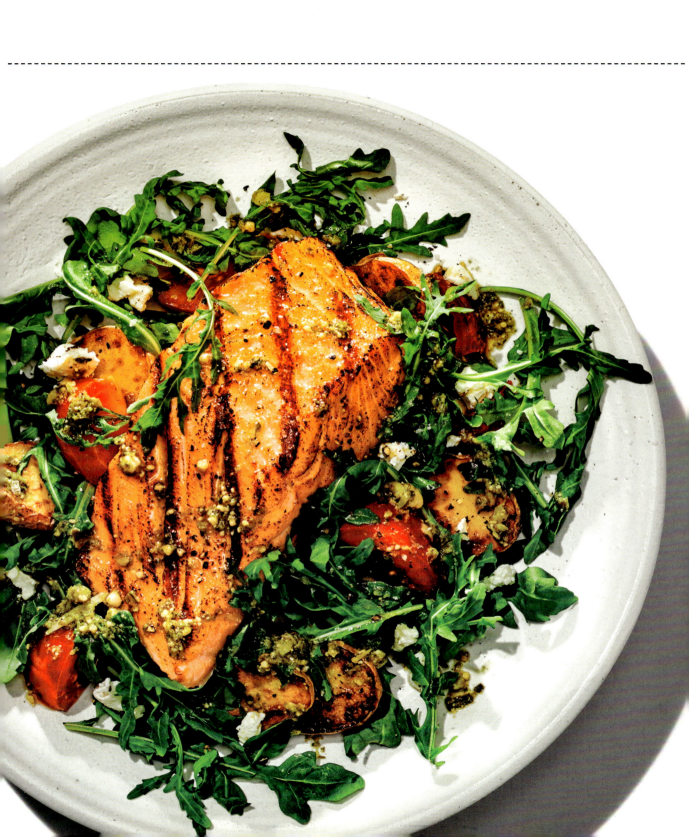

MH BEST MEALS FOR MUSCLE

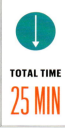

TOTAL TIME
25 MIN

CHICKEN MOLE TACOS

WHAT YOU'LL NEED

- ¾ LB CHICKEN BREAST
- ¾ TSP COCOA POWDER
- ¾ TSP ANCHO CHILI POWDER
- ½ TSP CINNAMON
- KOSHER SALT AND PEPPER
- ½ RED ONION, DICED
- ½ RED BELL PEPPER, DICED
- 1 SMALL RED CABBAGE, DICED
- 1 TBSP LIME JUICE
- 4 CORN TORTILLAS

HOW TO MAKE IT

▶ Preheat oven to 425°F. Line a rimmed baking sheet with foil. In medium bowl, toss chicken with cocoa powder, chili powder, cinnamon, and ⅛ tsp each salt and pepper. Transfer chicken to prepared sheet and roast until cooked through, about 12 minutes.

▶ In large bowl, combine onion, bell pepper, and cabbage, and toss with lime juice and ⅛ tsp each salt and pepper.

▶ Warm tortillas, then fill with chicken and top with slaw.

MAKES 2 SERVINGS.

NUTRITION PER SERVING
360 CALORIES | **39 G PROTEIN** | **38 G CARBOHYDRATES (7 G FIBER)** | **6 G FAT**

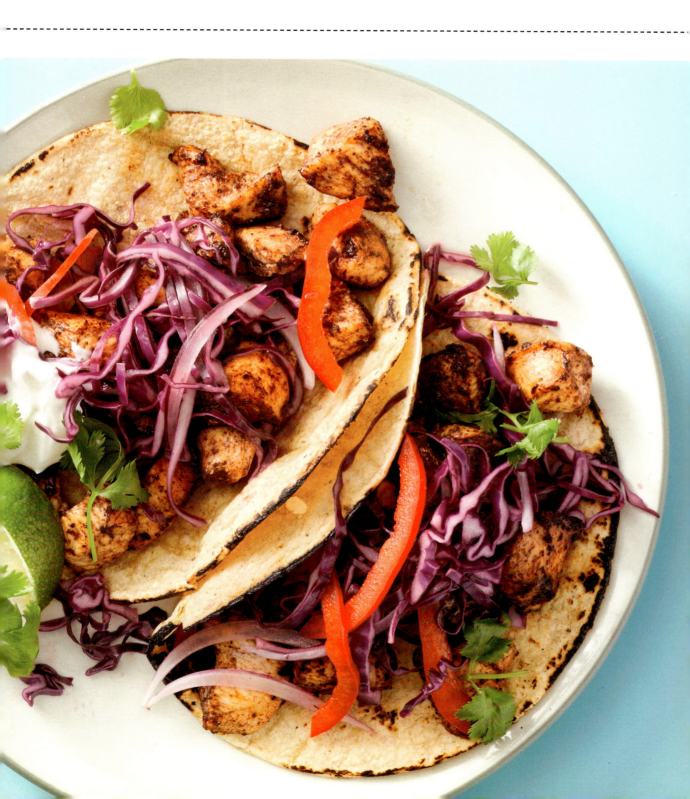

MH BEST MEALS FOR MUSCLE

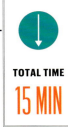

**TOTAL TIME
15 MIN**

MUSTARD MAPLE PORK CHOPS

WHAT YOU'LL NEED

- 1 TBSP MAPLE SYRUP
- 1 TBSP DIJON MUSTARD
- 1 TSP OLIVE OIL
- 1 SMALL CLOVE GARLIC, CRUSHED
- KOSHER SALT AND BLACK PEPPER TO TASTE
- 2 BONE-IN PORK CHOPS

HOW TO MAKE IT

▶ Heat cast-iron skillet over medium high. In small bowl, stir together the maple syrup, mustard, oil, garlic, salt, and pepper. Place mustard mixture and pork chops inside a large resealable plastic bag, and shake thoroughly to coat chops. Transfer chops to skillet, cooking about 3 minutes each side. In the last minute of cooking, pour remaining mustard mixture over chops.

MAKES 2 SERVINGS.

NUTRITION PER SERVING
282 CALORIES | 39 G PROTEIN | 9 G CARBOHYDRATES (0 G FIBER) | 9 G FAT

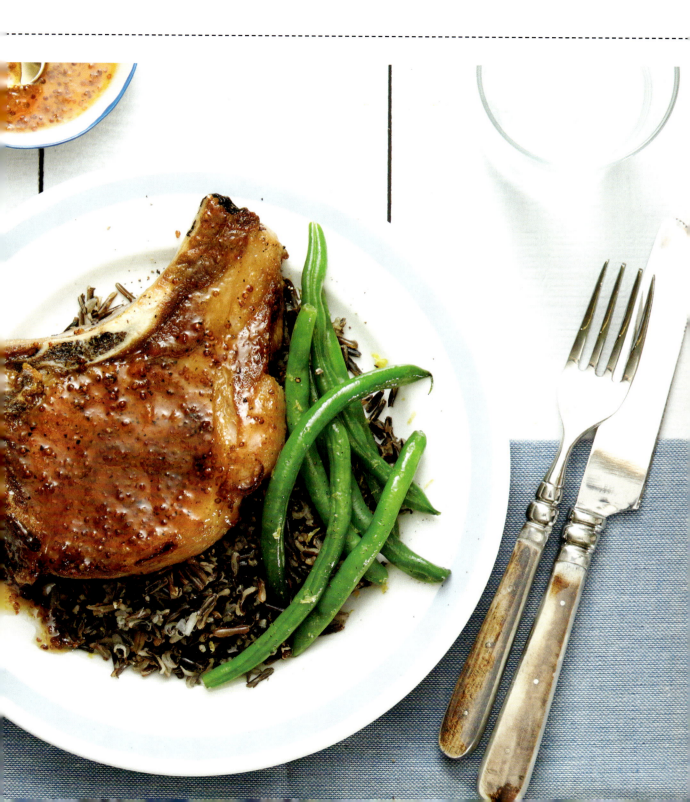

MH BEST MEALS FOR MUSCLE

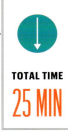

TOTAL TIME
25 MIN

LIME TILAPIA
with Citrus-Avocado Salsa

WHAT YOU'LL NEED

- ½ CUP WHITE RICE
- ½ TBSP LIME JUICE
- ½ TSP HONEY
- KOSHER SALT AND PEPPER
- ½ JALAPEÑO, THINLY SLICED
- 1 SCALLION, SLICED
- ½ ORANGE
- ½ GRAPEFRUIT
- ½ AVOCADO
- 2 SMALL TILAPIA FILLETS (about ⅞ lb total)
- 1 TBSP OLIVE OIL

HOW TO MAKE IT

▶ Cook rice according to package directions. In large bowl, whisk together lime juice, honey, and ⅛ tsp salt. Stir in jalapeño and white parts of scallions.

▶ Peel orange and grapefruit, and remove pith. Cut each into small pieces and add to bowl along with avocado; gently toss to combine.

▶ Heat a large skillet over medium high. Season tilapia with ¼ tsp each salt and pepper. Add 1 Tbsp oil to skillet and cook fillets until golden brown, about 4 minutes. Flip and cook until opaque throughout, 1 to 2 minutes. Transfer to plate.

▶ Serve fish over rice. Top with salsa and sprinkle with green parts of scallions.

MAKES 2 SERVINGS.

NUTRITION PER SERVING
535 CALORIES | 45 G PROTEIN | 57 G CARBOHYDRATES (6 G FIBER) | 16 G FAT

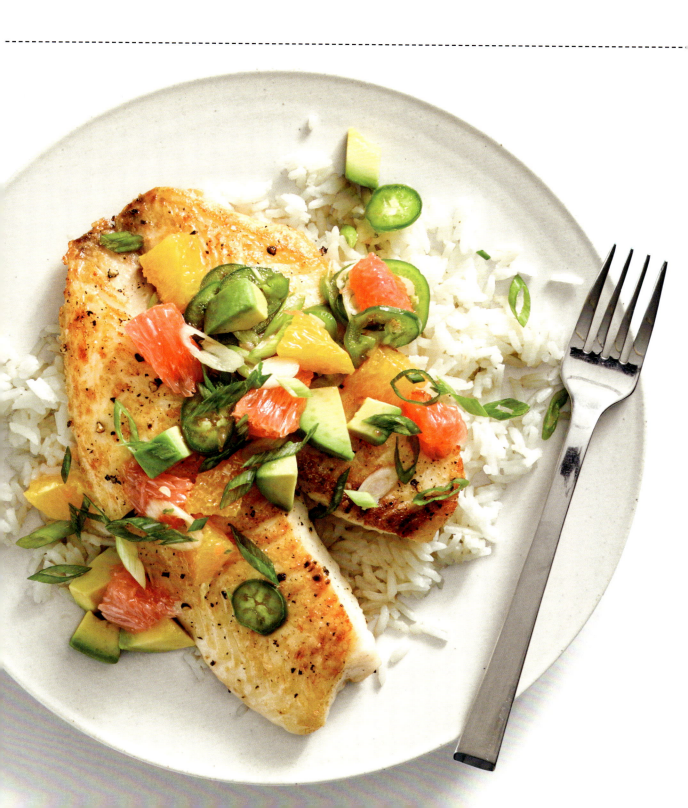

MH BEST MEALS FOR MUSCLE

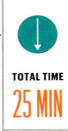

TOTAL TIME
25 MIN

SEARED SALMON
with Roasted Cauliflower

WHAT YOU'LL NEED

- 1½ LBS CAULIFLOWER FLORETS (about 1 large cauliflower head)
- 2 TBSP AND 2 TSP OLIVE OIL, DIVIDED
- KOSHER SALT AND PEPPER
- 4 6-OZ PIECES SALMON
- 2 CLOVES GARLIC, MINCED
- 1 TBSP CAPERS
- ½ CUP PARSLEY LEAVES

HOW TO MAKE IT

▶ Preheat oven to 450°F. In small bowl, toss cauliflower with 2 Tbsp oil and ¼ tsp salt and ¼ tsp pepper. Roast on baking sheet until tender, then broil until golden brown.

▶ Season salmon. Heat large skillet over medium high. Add 2 tsp oil to skillet and cook salmon until opaque throughout, about 5 minutes. Add garlic and capers to skillet after flipping the salmon.

▶ Toss cauliflower with garlic, capers, and parsley; serve with salmon.

MAKES 2 SERVINGS.

NUTRITION PER SERVING
608 CALORIES | **54 G PROTEIN** | **19 G CARBOHYDRATES (8 G FIBER)** | **36 G FAT**

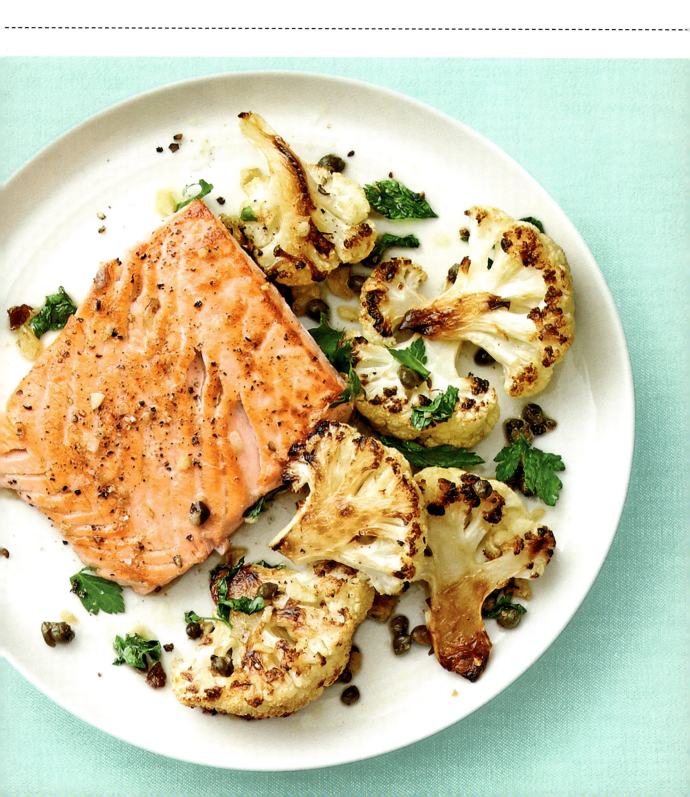

MH BEST MEALS FOR MUSCLE

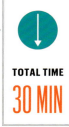

TOTAL TIME
30 MIN

SAUSAGE AND BROCCOLI RABE PASTA

WHAT YOU'LL NEED

- 1 LB BROCCOLI RABE, 2 IN. TRIMMED FROM ENDS, CUT IN 2-IN. PIECES
- 4 OZ PASTA
- 1 TBSP OLIVE OIL
- 6 OZ CHICKEN SAUSAGE, CUT IN ½-IN. SLICES
- 4 DRY-PACKED SUN-DRIED TOMATOES, ROUGHLY CHOPPED
- 3 CLOVES GARLIC, MINCED

HOW TO MAKE IT

▸ Heat large pot of water to boiling. Add the broccoli rabe and blanch for 2 minutes. Remove from pot with slotted spoon and plunge into cold water (save pot of hot water for pasta). Drain and set aside.

▸ Add pasta to boiling water. Stir and cook 10 minutes, or until al dente. Drain pasta, reserving 2 Tbsp cooking water.

▸ Heat oil in large skillet over medium high. Add sausage and cook, turning occasionally, for 5 minutes or until browned. Add the tomatoes, garlic, and broccoli rabe to skillet and cook until the sausage is no longer pink, about 2 minutes.

▸ Add pasta and reserved water to skillet. Toss with the sausage mixture.

MAKES 2 SERVINGS.

NUTRITION PER SERVING
470 CALORIES | 31 G PROTEIN | 53 G CARBOHYDRATES (9 G FIBER) | 16 G FAT

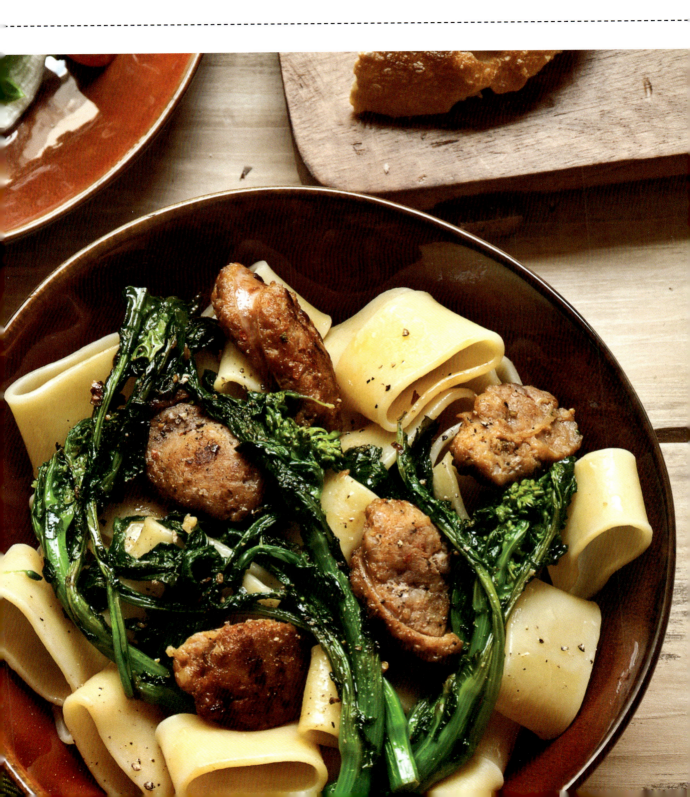

BEST MEALS FOR MUSCLE

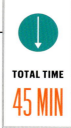

TOTAL TIME
45 MIN

ORANGE SWEET POTATO SALAD
with Chicken

WHAT YOU'LL NEED

- 2 LARGE SWEET POTATOES, CUBED
- 6 OZ COOKED CHICKEN, SLICED
- 4 TBSP OLIVE OIL, DIVIDED
- KOSHER SALT AND PEPPER
- 2 SLICES THICK BACON
- 1 RED BELL PEPPER, CHOPPED
- 1 SMALL RED ONION, HALVED AND THINLY SLICED
- 1 TBSP FRESH GINGER, MINCED
- 1 TSP GROUND CUMIN
- JUICE OF 1 ORANGE
- 1 LB SPINACH LEAVES

HOW TO MAKE IT

▶ Preheat oven to 400°F. Place sweet potatoes on baking sheet, drizzle with 2 Tbsp oil, sprinkle with ¾ tsp salt, and toss to coat. Roast, turning occasionally, until crisp and fork-tender, about 30 minutes. Remove from oven but leave on sheet until ready to use.

▶ While sweet potatoes roast, fry bacon in skillet over medium, turning once or twice, until crisp. Remove bacon and pour off fat, leaving any darkened bits in skillet. Chop the bacon. Heat skillet over medium and add remaining 2 Tbsp oil. Add bell pepper, onion, ginger, and ¼ teaspoon salt. Cook, stirring once or twice, until vegetables are tender. Stir in cumin and bacon. Add orange juice, and turn off heat.

▶ Put spinach in large bowl. Top with sweet potatoes, chicken, and warm dressing. (Note: If saving leftovers, only dress what you will eat immediately.) Toss to combine. Add salt and pepper to taste.

MAKES 2 SERVINGS.

NUTRITION PER SERVING

614 CALORIES | 40 G PROTEIN | 52 G CARBOHYDRATES (12 G FIBER) | 29 G FAT

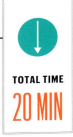

TOTAL TIME
20 MIN

VEGETARIAN STIR-FRY

WHAT YOU'LL NEED

- 1   12-OZ BLOCK TOFU, CUBED
- 1   TSP MINCED FRESH GINGER
- 2   CLOVES GARLIC, MINCED
- ¼   CUP CHOPPED CARROTS
- ¼   CUP CHOPPED ONION
- ¼   CUP CHOPPED BELL PEPPER
- ½   CUP CHOPPED MUSHROOMS
- ½   CUP CHOPPED BROCCOLI
- 2   TBSP LOW-SODIUM SOY SAUCE
- 1   CUP COOKED BROWN RICE

HOW TO MAKE IT

▶ Heat medium skillet over medium. Press tofu to remove excess water, and cut into 1-in. cubes. Add tofu to skillet and sauté with ginger and garlic, about 1 minute. Add vegetables. The water from tofu and vegetables will steam the mixture. Add a few tablespoons water, if needed. Cook until tofu is warm and vegetables are tender.

▶ Stir in the soy sauce and serve the stir-fry immediately with the rice.

MAKES 1 SERVING.

NUTRITION PER SERVING
587 CALORIES | 45 G PROTEIN | 66 G CARBOHYDRATES (11 G FIBER) | 20 G FAT

BONUS
Recipes

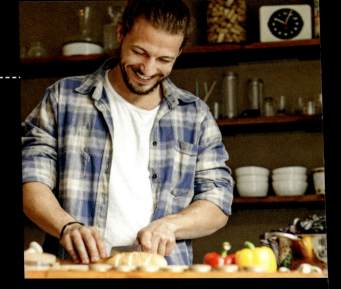

Work these meals into your plan however feels best for you. White recommends eating the lower-calorie meals before workouts and saving the heartier meals for after to most efficiently fuel the muscle-building process.

BREAKFASTS

- 83 SMOKED SALMON AND SCRAMBLED EGGS ON TOAST
- 84 BACON AND EGG FRIED RICE
- 86 RICOTTA AND LOX BREAKFAST BURRITO
- 87 BROCCOLI SPEARS OMELET
- 88 BEST-EVER SHAKSHUKA
- 90 SPINACH, EGG, AND CHEESE SANDWICH
- 91 GREEN EGGS AND HAM

LUNCHES

- 92 CHICKEN AVOCADO TACOS
- 93 SWEET ONION SALMON SALAD
- 94 TURKEY SLIDERS
- 96 JERK CHICKEN WITH CUCUMBER MANGO SALAD
- 98 SALMON BLT WITH HERBED SPREAD
- 100 MISO EGGPLANT GRAIN BOWL
- 102 TUNA TACOS
- 103 CARNITAS BURRITO BOWL
- 104 SWEET AND STICKY TOFU
- 106 CHEESY BLACK BEANS AND GREENS

DINNERS

- 107 QUINOA-STUFFED BELL PEPPERS
- 108 POTSTICKER AND VEGETABLE STIR-FRY
- 110 SPICY PORK FAJITAS
- 111 SUNDRIED TOMATO AND FETA BAKED CHICKEN
- 112 PAPRIKA CHICKEN WITH CRISPY CHICKPEAS AND TOMATOES
- 114 HERBED MOJO STEAK AND CRISPY POTATOES
- 116 SHEET PAN CHICKPEA CHICKEN
- 118 CHILI MANGO CHICKEN
- 119 SWEET AND SOUR PORK
- 120 FRESH VEGGIE BEEF RAGU
- 122 SALMON TERIYAKI WITH ASPARAGUS
- 123 SMOKY AND SPICY SAUSAGE HEROES
- 124 SPICED MEATBALL PITAS WITH CRISPY COLE SLAW

BREAKFAST

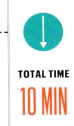

TOTAL TIME
10 MIN

SMOKED SALMON AND SCRAMBLED EGGS ON TOAST

WHAT YOU'LL NEED

- 2 SLICES WHOLE WHEAT BREAD
- 2 EGGS
- SALT AND GROUND BLACK PEPPER
- 1 OZ SLICED SMOKED SALMON
- THINLY SLICED RED ONION, CAPERS, CHOPPED FRESH DILL, AND/OR A LEMON WEDGE, FOR SERVING

HOW TO MAKE IT

▶ Toast the bread. Meanwhile, in a bowl, whisk the eggs with salt and pepper. Pour the eggs into a nonstick pan and scramble them. Lay the smoked salmon on the toast; top that with the scrambled egg. Finish with your choice of red onion, capers, fresh dill, and/or a squeeze of lemon.

MAKES 1 SERVING.

Meal Maker
Eat with ¼ medium avocado.

NUTRITION PER SERVING
480 CALORIES | 38 G PROTEIN | 29 G CARBOHYDRATES (4 G FIBER) | 22 G FAT

MH BEST MEALS FOR MUSCLE

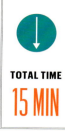

TOTAL TIME
15 MIN

BACON AND EGG FRIED RICE

WHAT YOU'LL NEED

- 1 TBSP CANOLA OIL
- 5 SLICES BACON, CHOPPED
- 1 BUNCH GREEN ONIONS, SLICED
- 1 (5-oz) BAG BABY SPINACH
- 3 CUPS COOKED WHITE RICE
- 1 CUP FROZEN PEAS
- ½ TSP SALT
- 8 FRIED EGGS

HOW TO MAKE IT

▶ In a 12-in. skillet, heat canola oil on medium-high. Add bacon and cook until bacon is crisp.

▶ Add green onions and baby spinach. Cook for 2 minutes, stirring.

▶ Add white rice, frozen peas, and salt. Cook for 5 minutes, stirring.

▶ Divide among 4 plates; top each with 2 fried eggs.

MAKES 4 SERVINGS.

NUTRITION PER SERVING
522 CALORIES, 23 G PROTEIN, 42 G CARBOHYDRATES (3 G FIBER), 32 G FAT

BREAKFAST

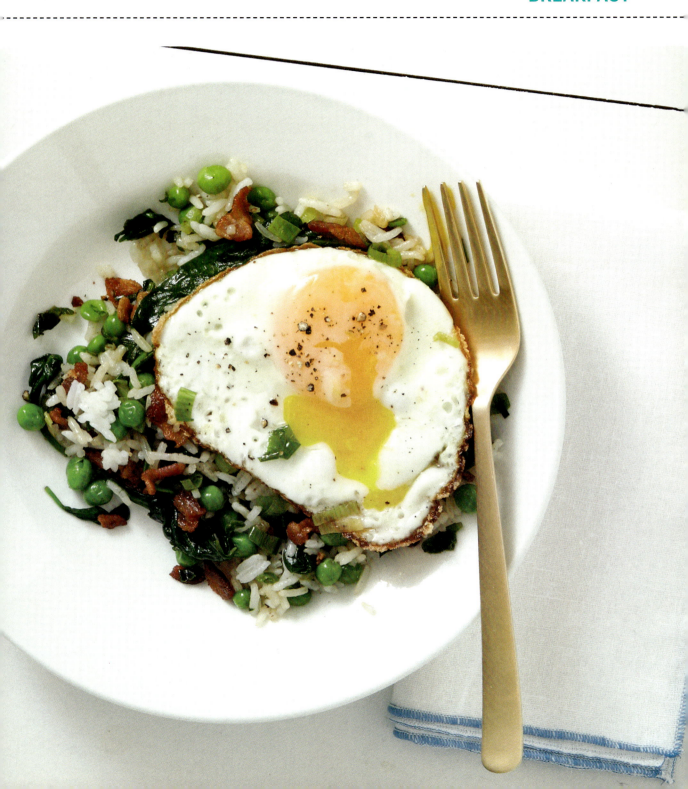

MH BEST MEALS FOR MUSCLE

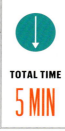

TOTAL TIME
5 MIN

RICOTTA AND LOX BREAKFAST BURRITO

WHAT YOU'LL NEED

- 2 TBSP RICOTTA CHEESE
- 1 MEDIUM WHOLE WHEAT TORTILLA
- 1 OZ SMOKED SALMON, TORN INTO LITTLE PIECES
- 2 EGGS, SCRAMBLED IN A NONSTICK PAN
- 1 CUP BABY SPINACH, CHOPPED
- 1 GREEN ONION, SLICED

HOW TO MAKE IT

▶ Spread the cheese on the tortilla, then arrange the salmon, eggs, spinach, and green onions on top. Fold the ends in, roll, and enjoy.

MAKES 1 SERVING.

Meal Maker
Eat with ¼ medium avocado and 1 serving of fruit.

NUTRITION PER SERVING
372 CALORIES | 38 G PROTEIN | 25 G CARBOHYDRATES (3 G FIBER) | 16 G FAT

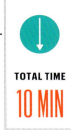

BREAKFAST

TOTAL TIME
10 MIN

BROCCOLI SPEARS OMELET

WHAT YOU'LL NEED

- 5 LARGE EGGS
- ½ HANDFUL OF FRESH PARSLEY, CHOPPED
- SPLASH OF SOY SAUCE
- 2 TSP OLIVE OIL
- 2 TBSP BROCCOLI FLORETS
- 5 SPEARS ASPARAGUS, CHOPPED
- ¼ CUP STRING BEANS, HALVED
- ½ CUP SPINACH
- 1 CLOVE GARLIC, CHOPPED
- DASH OF GROUND BLACK PEPPER

HOW TO MAKE IT

- ▶ Mix the eggs, parsley, and soy sauce in a bowl.
- ▶ Coat a skillet with the olive oil and sauté the broccoli, asparagus, beans, spinach, garlic, and black pepper for 5 minutes.
- ▶ Pour the egg mixture over the vegetables. Stir it for about 30 seconds and then let it sit for 1 minute. Stir it again until the eggs firm up and then let it sit for another minute. Then fold it and remove it from the pan.

MAKES 2 SERVINGS.

Meal Maker
Eat with 2 slices of whole grain toast and 1 cup of fruit.

NUTRITION PER SERVING
223 CALORIES | 15 G PROTEIN | 5 G CARBOHYDRATES (2 G FIBER) | 14 G FAT

MH BEST MEALS FOR MUSCLE

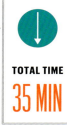

TOTAL TIME
35 MIN

BEST-EVER SHAKSHUKA

WHAT YOU'LL NEED

- 2 TBSP OLIVE OIL
- 1 YELLOW ONION, FINELY CHOPPED
- 1 CLOVE GARLIC, FINELY CHOPPED
- 1 TSP GROUND CUMIN
- KOSHER SALT AND GROUND BLACK PEPPER
- 1 LB TOMATOES, HALVED IF LARGE
- 8 LARGE EGGS
- ¼ CUP BABY SPINACH, FINELY CHOPPED
- ⅛ TOASTED BAGUETTE, FOR SERVING

HOW TO MAKE IT

- Preheat oven to 400°F. Heat oil in large oven-safe skillet on medium. Add onion and sauté until golden brown and tender, 8 minutes.
- Stir in garlic, cumin and ½ tsp each salt and pepper and cook 1 minute.
- Stir in tomatoes, transfer to oven and roast 10 minutes.
- Stir, then make 8 small wells in vegetable mixture and carefully crack 1 egg into each. Bake eggs to desired doneness, 7 to 8 minutes for slightly runny yolks. Sprinkle with spinach and serve with toast.

MAKES 2 SERVINGS.

NUTRITION PER SERVING
538 CALORIES | 30 G PROTEIN | 29 G CARBOHYDRATES (5 G FIBER) | 34 G FAT

BREAKFAST

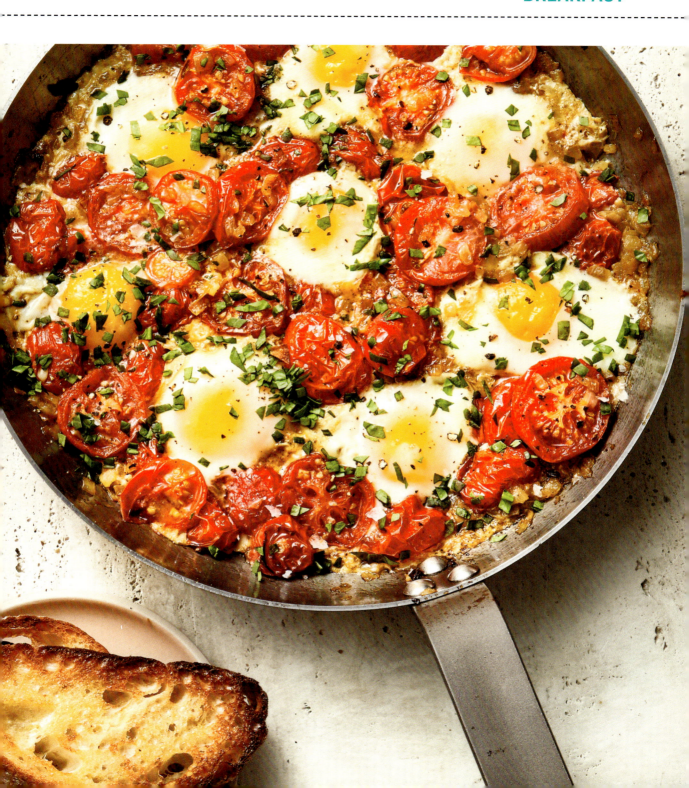

MH BEST MEALS FOR MUSCLE

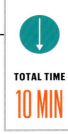

TOTAL TIME
10 MIN

SPINACH, EGG, AND CHEESE SANDWICH

WHAT YOU'LL NEED

- 1 (1-oz) SLICE BACON
- ½ TSP EXTRA-VIRGIN OLIVE OIL
- 1 EGG
- 1 MULTIGRAIN ENGLISH MUFFIN, TOASTED
- 1½ OZ (about 1 cup, packed) TRIMMED SPINACH LEAVES OR BABY SPINACH
- ½ TSP FRESHLY GROUND BLACK PEPPER
- 1 SLICE SWISS, JARLSBERG, OR HAVARTI CHEESE

HOW TO MAKE IT

▶ Cook bacon slice per package directions.

▶ Heat the oil in a small skillet over medium heat. Add the egg and heat it until the edges begin to set, about 1 minute. Lift the edges to allow any uncooked egg to flow underneath. When it's almost set, gently flip the egg. Cook another minute, then transfer to the bottom half of the muffin and top with the bacon.

▶ Return the pan to the heat, add the spinach, and cook, stirring until it's wilted, about 1 minute. Place the spinach on top of the bacon, season with the pepper, add the cheese, and top with the other muffin half.

MAKES 1 SERVING.

Meal Maker
Eat with 1 serving of fruit.

NUTRITION PER SERVING (COMPUTED WITH SWISS CHEESE)
462 G CALORIES | 23 G PROTEIN | 29 G CARBOHYDRATES (2 G FIBER) | 28 G FAT

BREAKFAST

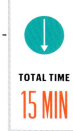

TOTAL TIME
15 MIN

GREEN EGGS AND HAM

WHAT YOU'LL NEED

- 1 TBSP DISTILLED WHITE VINEGAR
- 8 EGGS
- 2 TBSP PREPARED PESTO
- 2 TBSP PLAIN GREEK YOGURT
- 4 WHOLE WHEAT ENGLISH MUFFINS, SPLIT
- 4–8 SLICES HAM, PROSCIUTTO, OR COOKED CANADIAN BACON
- ¼ CUP SLICED JARRED ROASTED RED PEPPERS
- SALT AND GROUND BLACK PEPPER

HOW TO MAKE IT

▶ Bring 3 in. of water to a boil in a large skillet or wide saucepan. Reduce to a bare simmer and add the vinegar. Working in two batches, poach the eggs until the whites are just firm, 3 to 5 minutes. Using a slotted spoon, remove the eggs to a plate.

▶ In a small bowl, mix together the pesto and yogurt until they're smooth and combined. Toast the split English muffins until golden.

▶ Dividing evenly, top 4 of the muffin halves with the ham, roasted peppers, and eggs. Season with salt and black pepper to taste and add the pesto mixture. Top the eggs with the remaining muffin halves.

MAKES 4 SERVINGS.

Meal Maker
Eat with 1 cup of fruit.

NUTRITION PER SERVING
363 CALORIES | 24 G PROTEIN | 31 G CARBOHYDRATES (5 G FIBER) | 17 G FAT

MH BEST MEALS FOR MUSCLE

CHICKEN AVOCADO TACOS

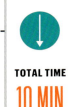

**TOTAL TIME
10 MIN**

WHAT YOU'LL NEED

- 1½ TSP CANOLA OIL
- 3 CORN TORTILLAS (6-in. diameter)
- ¼ AVOCADO, SLICED
- 1½ OZ SKINLESS CHICKEN BREAST, COOKED AND THINLY SLICED
- ½ CUP BLACK BEANS, RINSED AND DRAINED
- 1½ LEAVES LETTUCE, SHREDDED
- 3 TSP STORE-BOUGHT SALSA
- 3 TSP FRESH CILANTRO, MINCED

HOW TO MAKE IT

▶ Heat the oil in a skillet over medium-high heat. Cook the tortillas for about 1 minute on each side, or until lightly browned (they will become crisp as they cool).

▶ Transfer the tortillas to a work surface. Place the avocado across the 3 tortillas. Top each with the chicken, black beans, lettuce, salsa, and cilantro.

MAKES 1 SERVING.

NUTRITION PER SERVING
498 CALORIES | 27 G PROTEIN | 60 G CARBOHYDRATES (17 G FIBER) | 18 G FAT

SWEET ONION SALMON SALAD

LUNCH

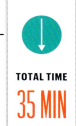

TOTAL TIME
35 MIN

WHAT YOU'LL NEED

- 2 SALMON FILLETS (6 OZ EACH), RINSED AND DRIED
- 1 TSP DRIED OR FRESH PARSLEY
- JUICE OF ½ LEMON
- 1 TSP GROUND BLACK PEPPER + 1 PINCH, DIVIDED
- 4 CUPS SPINACH LEAVES
- 10 GRAPE OR CHERRY TOMATOES, HALVED
- ½ CUP BLUEBERRIES
- 1 TSP EXTRA-VIRGIN OLIVE OIL
- ½ CUP SWEET ONION, CHOPPED
- 1 CLOVE GARLIC, MINCED
- 20 ASPARAGUS SPEARS, BOTTOMS CUT OFF
- ½ YELLOW BELL PEPPER, CUT INTO STRIPS
- 1 TBSP HONEY MUSTARD
- 1 TBSP ALMONDS, SLIVERED

HOW TO MAKE IT

- Place the salmon in a deep skillet big enough for the salmon to lie flat on the bottom. Cover the fish with 1 in. of water.
- Add the parsley, lemon juice, and 1 tsp of black pepper.
- Bring to a boil over medium heat. Boil for 10 to 15 minutes, or until the fish is opaque.
- Lightly scrape off the skin and fat line.
- Evenly divide the spinach, tomato, and blueberries between two plates. Top each with half of the salmon.
- In another skillet, combine the oil, onion, and garlic. Cook over medium-high heat for 2 minutes, or until lightly browned.
- Add the asparagus, bell pepper, and a pinch of black pepper.
- Reduce the heat to medium. Cook for 2 to 3 minutes, or until the veggies are slightly tender.
- Add the honey mustard. Cook for 30 seconds longer, or until the honey mustard slightly caramelizes.
- Place the mixture over the salmon. Sprinkle with the almonds.

MAKES 2 SERVINGS.

Meal Maker
Eat with 1 cup of fruit.

NUTRITION PER SERVING
496 CALORIES | 42 G PROTEIN | 33 G CARBOHYDRATES | (10 G FIBER) | 23 G FAT

MH BEST MEALS FOR MUSCLE

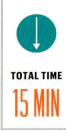

TOTAL TIME
15 MIN

TURKEY SLIDERS

WHAT YOU'LL NEED

- 1 EGG WHITE, BEATEN
- ½ SMALL RED ONION, MINCED
- ¼ CUP FRESH CILANTRO, MINCED
- ½ TSP GROUND CUMIN
- ¼ TSP SALT
- 1 LB EXTRA-LEAN GROUND TURKEY BREAST (99% fat-free)
- 8 WHOLE WHEAT DINNER ROLLS, CUT IN HALF
- 4 LEAVES LETTUCE, HALVED
- 2 PLUM TOMATOES, EACH CUT INTO 4 SLICES
- 1 AVOCADO, SLICED

SLICED ONION OR PICKLED HOT PEPPERS, FOR TOPPINGS IF DESIRED

HOW TO MAKE IT

▶ Whisk together the egg white, onion, cilantro, cumin, and salt in a medium bowl.

▶ Add the turkey and mix until just blended.

▶ Shape into 8 burgers, about 3 in. thick each.

▶ Heat a skillet coated with cooking spray over medium heat. Cook the burgers, turning once, for 6 minutes or until well browned and a thermometer inserted in the thickest portion registers 165°F.

▶ Place the bottoms of 2 dinner rolls on 4 plates. Top with 1 piece of lettuce and 1 tomato slice. Place 1 burger on each and top with the avocado and the top of the roll.

MAKES 4 SERVINGS.

Meal Maker
Eat with 2 cups of vegetables.

NUTRITION PER SERVING
432 CALORIES | 36 G PROTEIN | 48 G CARBOHYDRATES (10 G FIBER) | 13 G FAT

LUNCH

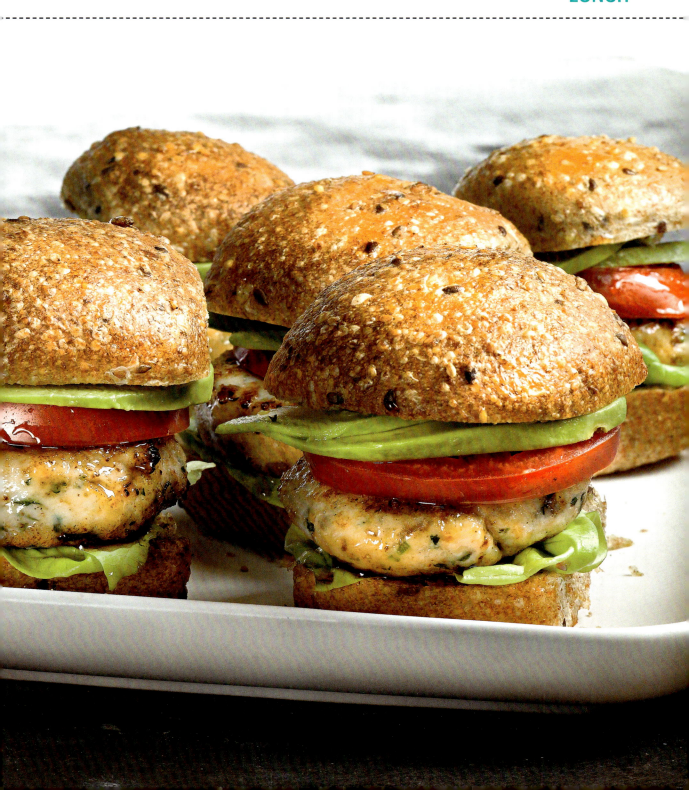

MH BEST MEALS FOR MUSCLE

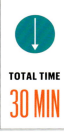

TOTAL TIME
30 MIN

JERK CHICKEN
With Cucumber Mango Salad

WHAT YOU'LL NEED

- ½ SMALL RED ONION, THINLY SLICED
- 2 TBSP FRESH LIME JUICE, PLUS LIME WEDGES FOR SERVING
- KOSHER SALT
- GROUND BLACK PEPPER
- 1 RIPE (but firm) MANGO, THINLY SLICED
- 1 SMALL SEEDLESS CUCUMBER, THINLY SLICED INTO HALF-MOONS
- 1 TBSP OLIVE OIL
- 1 TBSP SALT-FREE JERK SEASONING
- 8 THIN-CUT CHICKEN BREASTS (about 1½ lbs total)
- ¼ CUP CILANTRO, CHOPPED

HOW TO MAKE IT

- Heat grill or grill pan over medium. In a large bowl, toss onion, lime juice, and pinch each salt and pepper, then toss with mango and cucumber. Let sit, tossing occasionally, at least 10 minutes.
- Meanwhile, in a small bowl, combine oil, jerk seasoning, and ¼ tsp salt, then rub all over chicken. Grill until just cooked through, 2 to 4 minutes per side.
- Fold cilantro into cucumber salad and serve with chicken and lime wedges if desired.

MAKES 4 SERVINGS.

Meal Maker
Eat with ½ cup white rice and 1 cup vegetables.

NUTRITION PER SERVING
275 CALORIES | 36 G PROTEIN | 15 G CARBOHYDRATES (2 G FIBER) | 8 G FAT

LUNCH

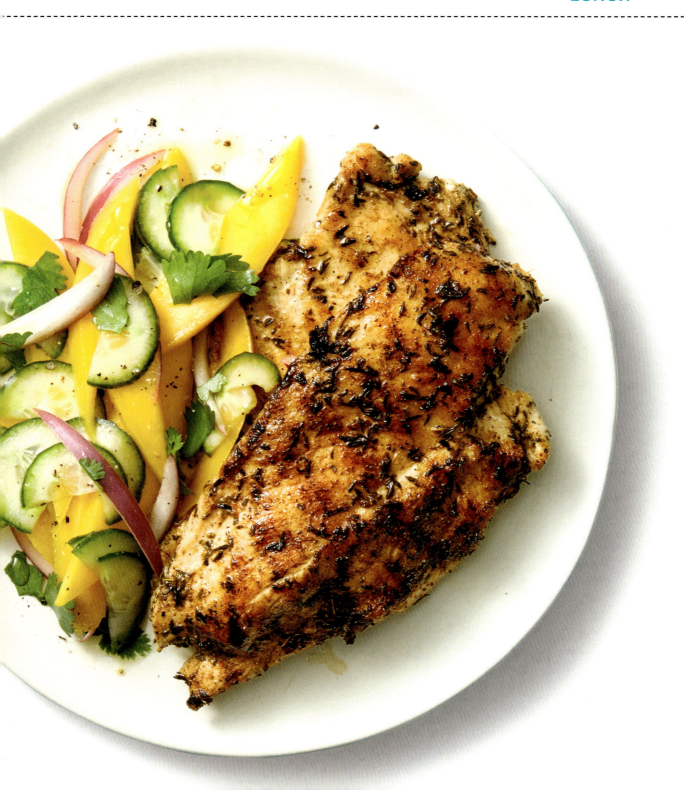

MH BEST MEALS FOR MUSCLE

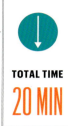

TOTAL TIME
20 MIN

SALMON BLT
with Herbed Spread

WHAT YOU'LL NEED

- 6 SLICES BACON
- ½ CUP PLAIN LOW-FAT GREEK YOGURT
- ¼ FRESH DILL, CHOPPED
- 1 GREEN ONION, CHOPPED
- KOSHER SALT AND GROUND BLACK PEPPER
- 1 TBSP OLIVE OIL
- 1 LB SKINLESS SALMON FILLET, CUT INTO 4 THIN PIECES
- 8 SLICES WHOLE GRAIN BREAD
- 4 LEAVES LETTUCE
- 1 TOMATO, SLICED

HOW TO MAKE IT

▶ Cook bacon until crisp. Transfer to a paper towel–lined plate; break into pieces when cool.

▶ Meanwhile, combine yogurt, dill, green onion, and ¼ tsp each salt and pepper.

▶ Heat oil in a large skillet on medium. Cook salmon until opaque throughout, 1 to 2 minutes per side.

▶ Spread yogurt mixture on bread and top 4 slices with lettuce, tomato, salmon, and bacon. Sandwich with remaining slices of bread.

MAKES 4 SERVINGS.

NUTRITION PER SERVING
494 CALORIES | 38 G PROTEIN | 50 G CARBOHYDRATES (3 G FIBER) | 15 G FAT

LUNCH

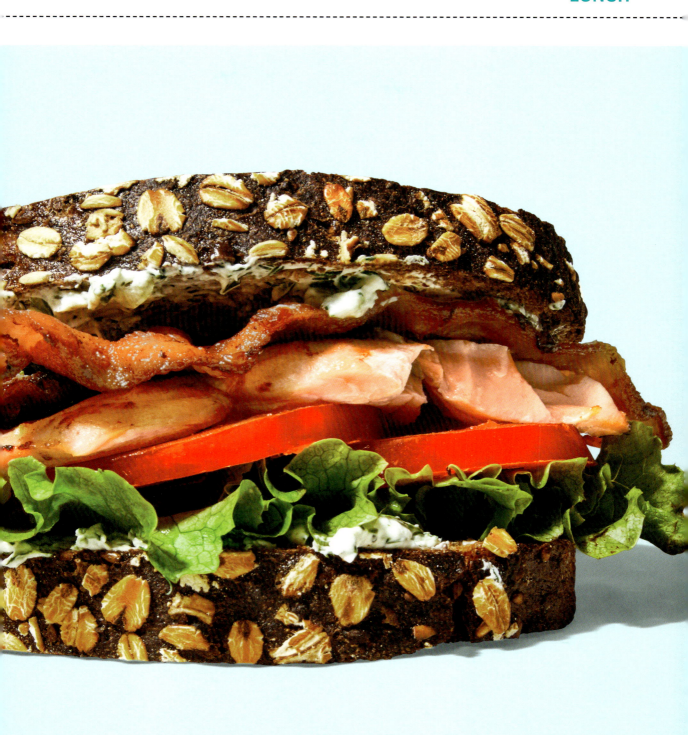

MH BEST MEALS FOR MUSCLE

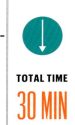

TOTAL TIME
30 MIN

MISO EGGPLANT GRAIN BOWL

WHAT YOU'LL NEED

- ½ CUP QUINOA
- ¼ CUP PEARL BARLEY
- ¼ CUP LENTILS
- 1 TBSP WHITE MISO PASTE
- 2 TSP MIRIN
- 1 TBSP SOY SAUCE
- 2 TBSP CANOLA OIL
- 1 SMALL EGGPLANT, DICED
- 2 CUPS BROCCOLI FLORETS
- 2 TBSP SESAME DRESSING

FOR TOPPING (⅓ CUP EACH)
- DICED EXTRA-FIRM TOFU
- EDAMAME (thawed)
- DICED AVOCADO
- PICKLED RED CABBAGE
- THINLY SLICED CARROT

HOW TO MAKE IT

▶ In a medium pot, combine the quinoa, barley, lentils, and 1¾ cup water. Bring to a boil, uncovered, and then lower the heat to low. Put a lid on the pot and simmer until the grains are tender, 15 to 20 minutes.

▶ In a small bowl, whisk together the miso, mirin, soy sauce, and 1 tsp water. Set aside.

▶ In a large pan over medium, heat 1 Tbsp oil. Add the eggplant and cook until browned, 6 to 8 minutes. Add the reserved sauce and simmer until saucy, 2 minutes. Transfer to a plate.

▶ Wipe out the pan, add the remaining oil, and return it to medium heat. Add the broccoli and sauté until tender, about 3 minutes. Season with salt. Transfer to the plate with the eggplant.

▶ Toss the grains with the dressing and divide it among 3 bowls. Top each with reserved eggplant and broccoli, plus any toppings, if desired.

MAKES 3 SERVINGS.

NUTRITION PER SERVING
652 CALORIES | 29 G PROTEIN | 92 G CARBOHYDRATES (23 G FIBER) | 21 G FAT

LUNCH

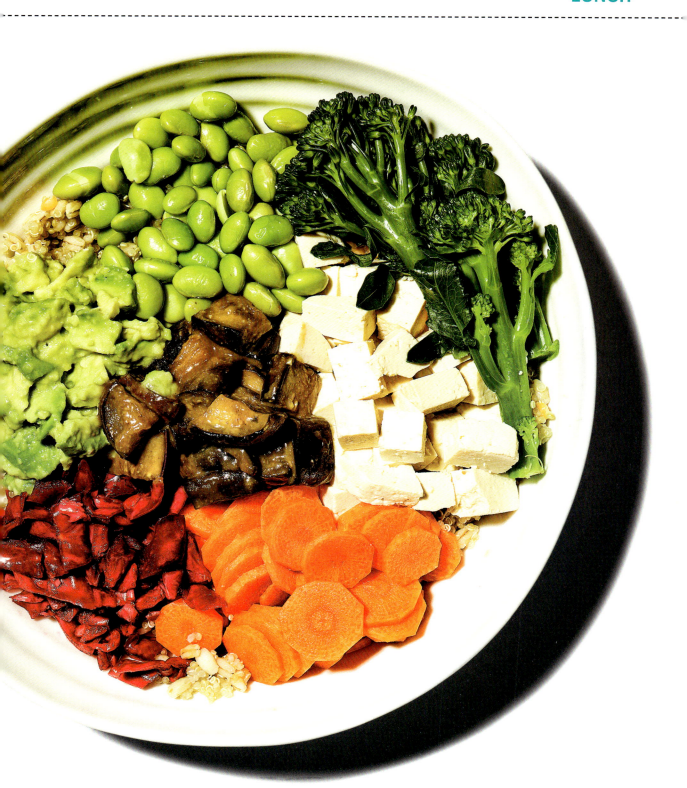

MH BEST MEALS FOR MUSCLE

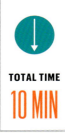

TOTAL TIME
10 MIN

TUNA TACOS

WHAT YOU'LL NEED

- 1   (5-oz) CAN TUNA, PACKED IN WATER, DRAINED
- 2   TBSP + 1 TSP LIME JUICE
- 2   TBSP MINCED RED ONION
- 1   TBSP CHOPPED MINT
- ½   TBSP OLIVE OIL
- ½   CUP SHREDDED RED CABBAGE
- ¼   CUP GRATED CARROTS
- 1   TBSP MINCED PICKLED JALAPEÑOS
- 2   WARM CORN TORTILLAS

HOW TO MAKE IT

▶ Mix the tuna, 2 Tbsp of the lime juice, onion, mint, and oil. Separately, combine the cabbage, carrots, and the jalapeños with the remaining 1 tsp lime juice.

▶ Top the tortillas with the tuna mixture, cabbage slaw, and more chopped mint.

MAKES 1 SERVING.

Meal Maker
Eat with 1 cup white rice.

NUTRITION PER SERVING
355 CALORIES | 31 G PROTEIN | 32 G CARBOHYDRATES (5 G FIBER) | 12 G FAT

LUNCH

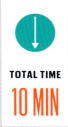

TOTAL TIME
10 MIN

CARNITAS BURRITO BOWL

WHAT YOU'LL NEED

- ½ CUP SHREDDED PORK, CHOPPED
- ¼ MEDIUM AVOCADO
- 2 TBSP SOUR CREAM
- 1 TBSP LIME JUICE
- 2 CUPS MIXED GREENS
- ½ CUP COOKED BROWN RICE
- ½ CUP CANNED BLACK BEANS, RINSED AND DRAINED
- 1 PLUM TOMATO, CHOPPED
- ½ SMALL RED ONION, THINLY SLICED

HOW TO MAKE IT

▶ Heat a small, oiled nonstick skillet on medium. Add the pork and cook until it's crisped in places, about 3 minutes.

▶ In a blender or food processor, puree the avocado, sour cream, and lime juice, adding water 1 Tbsp at a time until the dressing is the right consistency for drizzling. Season with salt and pepper.

▶ Add the greens to a bowl and top with the rice, beans, tomato, onion, and pork. Finish with a drizzle of the avocado dressing.

MAKES 1 SERVING.

NUTRITION PER SERVING
646 CALORIES | **32 G PROTEIN** | **57 G CARBOHYDRATES (13 G FIBER)** | **33 G FAT**

MH BEST MEALS FOR MUSCLE

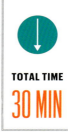

TOTAL TIME
30 MIN

SWEET AND STICKY TOFU

WHAT YOU'LL NEED

- 4 OZ UDON NOODLES
- 2 TBSP LOW-SODIUM SOY SAUCE
- 1 TSP BROWN SUGAR
- 1 TSP CORNSTARCH
- GROUND BLACK PEPPER
- 1 (14-oz) PACKAGE FIRM TOFU, DRAINED
- 2 TBSP CANOLA OIL
- 2 CLOVES GARLIC, FINELY CHOPPED
- 1 (1-in.) PIECE FRESH GINGER, PEELED AND CUT INTO MATCHSTICKS
- 4 GREEN ONIONS, THINLY SLICED
- 1 SMALL RED CHILE, THINLY SLICED
- 2 BUNCHES BABY BOK CHOY, LEAVES SEPARATED AND HALVED LENGTHWISE
- 2 CUPS BABY SPINACH

HOW TO MAKE IT

▶ Cook udon noodles per package directions. In a small bowl, combine ¼ cup water, soy sauce, brown sugar, cornstarch, and ½ tsp pepper until smooth.

▶ Blot tofu dry with paper towels. Cut into ¾-in. pieces. Heat a large skillet on medium-high. Add 1 Tbsp oil, then tofu, and cook, stirring occasionally, until golden brown, 6 to 8 minutes. Transfer to a plate; wipe out skillet.

▶ Add remaining Tbsp oil, then garlic, ginger, and half the green onions and chile and cook 1 minute. Add bok choy and cook, tossing, 2 minutes.

▶ Fold in tofu, then soy sauce mixture. Simmer until thickened, about 1 minute; toss with spinach. Spoon over cooked udon noodles and top with remaining green onions and chile.

MAKES 2 SERVINGS.

NUTRITION PER SERVING
457 CALORIES | 28 G PROTEIN | 36 G CARBOHYDRATES (6 G FIBER) | 25 G FAT

LUNCH

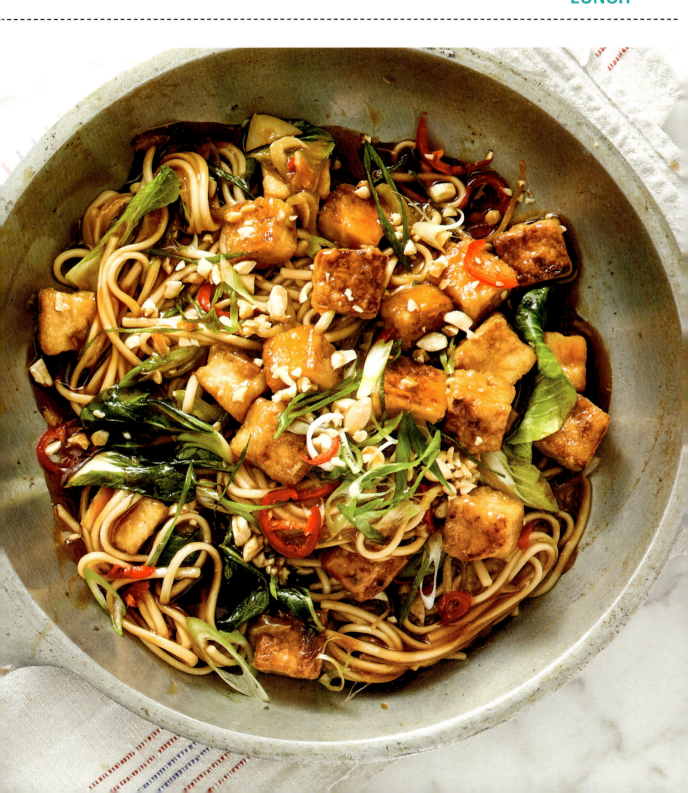

BEST MEALS FOR MUSCLE

LUNCH

CHEESY BLACK BEANS AND GREENS

TOTAL TIME
30 MIN

WHAT YOU'LL NEED

- 5 SOFT CORN TORTILLAS (6-in. diameter)
- 6 GREEN ONIONS, CHOPPED
- 1 RED BELL PEPPER, CHOPPED
- 1 SMALL JALAPEÑO PEPPER, SEEDED AND FINELY CHOPPED
- 1 CLOVE GARLIC, MINCED
- 1 TSP GROUND CUMIN
- 1 (15-oz) CAN REDUCED-SODIUM BLACK BEANS, RINSED AND DRAINED
- 4 CUPS (about 4 oz) BABY SPINACH
- 1 LARGE TOMATO, CHOPPED
- 1 CUP CHEDDAR CHEESE, SHREDDED
- 4 TBSP SOUR CREAM
- FRESH CILANTRO, CHOPPED, FOR GARNISH

HOW TO MAKE IT

▶ Preheat the oven to 350°F. Stack the tortillas on a large piece of foil, sprinkle the top one with water, and wrap them in the foil. Heat for 10 minutes.

▶ Meanwhile, heat a large skillet coated with olive oil cooking spray over medium-high heat. Add the green onions and bell pepper and cook for 5 minutes, or until lightly browned. Add the jalapeño pepper, garlic, and cumin. Cook for 2 minutes or until lightly browned. Stir in the beans, spinach, and tomato. Cook for 2 minutes or until heated through. Spread the mixture evenly in the skillet.

▶ Remove the mixture from the heat and sprinkle it with the cheese. Let it stand until the cheese is melted. Top with dollops of sour cream and sprinkle it with the cilantro.

▶ Cut the warmed tortillas into quarters or strips. Serve immediately with the cheesy bean-vegetable mixture.

MAKES 2 SERVINGS.

NUTRITION PER SERVING
671 CALORIES | 34 G PROTEIN | 79 G CARBOHYDRATES (24 G FIBER) | 27 G FAT

DINNER

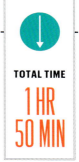

TOTAL TIME
1 HR 50 MIN

QUINOA-STUFFED BELL PEPPERS

WHAT YOU'LL NEED

- ⅓ CUP ALMONDS, SLIVERED
- ¼ TSP KOSHER SALT
- ¾ CUP QUINOA
- 4 LARGE RED, ORANGE, OR YELLOW BELL PEPPERS
- 1 TSP OLIVE OIL
- 1 MEDIUM ONION, CHOPPED
- 2 LARGE CLOVES GARLIC, MINCED
- 1 (10-oz) PACKAGE FRESH SPINACH, TOUGH STEMS REMOVED, TORN INTO LARGE PIECES
- ½ CUP FETA CHEESE, CRUMBLED
- ¼ CUP DRIED CURRANTS OR RAISINS
- 1 (14½-oz) CAN DICED TOMATOES
- 2 TBSP TOMATO PASTE
- ¼ TSP DRIED ITALIAN SEASONING

HOW TO MAKE IT

▶ Preheat the oven to 375°F. Cook the slivered almonds in a small nonstick skillet over medium heat, stirring often, for 3 to 4 minutes or until lightly toasted. Transfer to plate; let cool. Cook quinoa per package directions. Uncover and set aside when done.

▶ Bring a large pot of water to a boil. Cut off and reserve the tops of the peppers. Remove the seeds and ribs. Add the peppers and tops to the boiling water and cook for 5 minutes. Drain.

▶ In the same pot, heat the oil over medium heat. Add the onion and cook, stirring occasionally, for 6 minutes or until golden brown. Stir in the garlic. Remove 2 Tbsp of the onion mixture and set aside. Add the spinach to the pot and cook, stirring frequently, for 5 minutes or until wilted. Remove the pot from the heat. Add the feta, currants or raisins, almonds, and quinoa to the spinach mixture. Stir to combine.

▶ Arrange the peppers in a shallow baking dish. Spoon in the stuffing and replace the tops. Add ½ in. of water to the baking dish. Cover loosely with foil and bake for 40 to 45 minutes or until the peppers are tender.

▶ Meanwhile, in a saucepan, combine the tomatoes (with juice), tomato paste, Italian seasoning, and the reserved 2 Tbsp of the onion mixture. Bring to a boil. Reduce the heat, cover, and simmer for 30 minutes or until thickened. Spoon the sauce onto plates and top with the peppers.

MAKES 2 SERVINGS.

NUTRITION PER SERVING
774 CALORIES | 28 G PROTEIN | 125 G CARBOHYDRATES (22 G FIBER) | 24 G FAT

MH BEST MEALS FOR MUSCLE

POTSTICKER AND VEGETABLE STIR-FRY

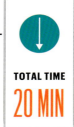

TOTAL TIME
20 MIN

WHAT YOU'LL NEED

- 2 TBSP CANOLA OIL
- 8 FROZEN PORK POTSTICKERS
- 1 TBSP REDUCED-SODIUM SOY SAUCE
- 1 TSP HONEY
- 3 MEDIUM CARROTS, THINLY SLICED ON A DIAGONAL
- 2 BELL PEPPERS (1 red, 1 yellow), THINLY SLICED
- 2 CLOVES GARLIC, FINELY CHOPPED
- 1 TBSP FINELY CHOPPED FRESH GINGER
- 1 MEDIUM RED ONION, THINLY SLICED
- ¼ MEDIUM GREEN CABBAGE, VERY THINLY SLICED (4 cups)
- 3 OZ SNOW PEAS, SLICED ON A DIAGONAL INTO THIRDS
- TOASTED SESAME SEEDS

HOW TO MAKE IT

▶ Heat 1 Tbsp oil in a large skillet over medium heat. Add the potstickers and cook until lightly browned on all sides, 4 to 6 minutes. Add 2 Tbsp water to the skillet, cover, and cook until the water has evaporated and the potstickers are heated through, 1 to 2 minutes. In a small bowl, whisk together the soy sauce and honey; set aside.

▶ Meanwhile, heat the remaining Tbsp oil in a large skillet over medium-high heat. Add the carrots, peppers, garlic, and ginger and cook, tossing occasionally, for 5 minutes. Add the onion, cabbage, and snow peas and cook, tossing occasionally, until the vegetables are just tender, about 2 minutes more.

▶ Divide the vegetables and potstickers among bowls and drizzle with the soy sauce mixture. Sprinkle with toasted sesame seeds, if desired.

MAKES 2 SERVINGS.

 NUTRITION PER SERVING
691 CALORIES | 23 G PROTEIN | 72 G CARBOHYDRATES (14 G FIBER) | 37 G FAT

DINNER

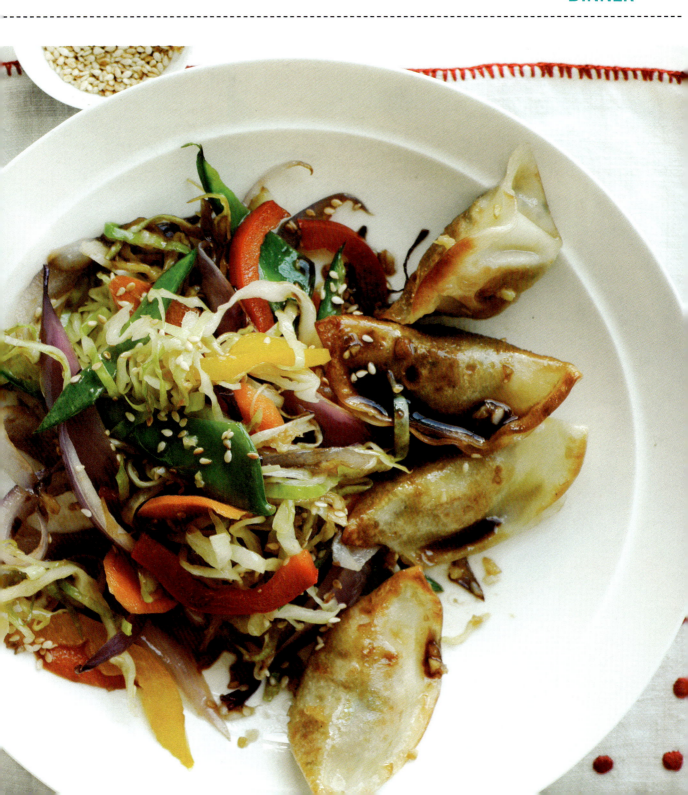

MH BEST MEALS FOR MUSCLE

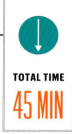

TOTAL TIME
45 MIN

SPICY PORK FAJITAS

WHAT YOU'LL NEED

- 1¼ LBS BONELESS PORK LOIN CHOPS, TRIMMED AND SLICED INTO ½-IN. STRIPS
- GRATED PEEL AND JUICE OF 1 LIME
- 3 CLOVES GARLIC, MINCED
- ½ TSP KOSHER SALT
- ¼ TSP CAYENNE PEPPER
- ¼ TSP GROUND BLACK PEPPER
- 4 TSP + 1 TBSP CANOLA OIL
- 3 LARGE BELL PEPPERS (mixed colors), SEEDED AND CUT INTO LONG, ½-IN.-THICK STRIPS
- 1 EXTRA-LARGE ONION, CUT INTO ½-IN.-THICK SLICES
- 2 JALAPEÑO PEPPERS, SEEDED AND CUT INTO THIN STRIPS
- 1 CUP CILANTRO LEAVES, TOUGH STEMS DISCARDED AND LOOSELY PACKED
- 12 FLOUR TORTILLAS, WARMED (6-in. diameter)

HOW TO MAKE IT

▶ Place the pork in a bowl with the lime zest, half of the lime juice, the garlic, salt, cayenne, black pepper, and 2 tsp of the oil. Toss to coat. Marinate the pork at room temperature for 20 minutes (or longer, or overnight in the fridge).

▶ Heat 1 Tbsp of oil in a wok (or 12-in. skillet) over medium-high heat. Add the bell peppers, onion, and jalapeño. Stir-fry until the onions and peppers are soft and slightly charred, 6 to 8 minutes. Transfer the peppers and onions to a metal bowl and toss with cilantro and the remaining lime juice. Cover with foil and keep warm.

▶ Return the wok to medium-high heat. Add the remaining 2 tsp of oil and the pork. Stir-fry until the meat is seared and just cooked through, 3 to 4 minutes. Place the pork in warmed tortillas and top with the vegetables.

MAKES 6 SERVINGS.

 NUTRITION PER SERVING
521 CALORIES | 29 G PROTEIN | 58 G CARBOHYDRATES (5 G FIBER) | 19 G FAT

SUNDRIED TOMATO AND FETA BAKED CHICKEN

DINNER

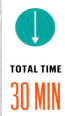

TOTAL TIME
30 MIN

WHAT YOU'LL NEED

- 2 TBSP JARRED SUN-DRIED TOMATOES, CHOPPED
- 2 TBSP FETA CHEESE, CRUMBLED
- 2 TBSP OLIVES, CHOPPED
- 2 GARLIC CLOVES, MINCED
- 1 TBSP BALSAMIC VINEGAR
- 2 BONELESS, SKINLESS CHICKEN BREASTS
- EXTRA-VIRGIN OLIVE OIL
- SALT AND GROUND BLACK PEPPER, TO TASTE
- 2 CUPS ORGANIC SPINACH

HOW TO MAKE IT

▸ Preheat the oven to 450°F. Toss together the tomatoes, feta cheese, olives, 1 clove of minced garlic, and vinegar.

▸ Rub the chicken with olive oil, salt, and pepper. Using a small, sharp knife, carefully cut a slit along the thick part of each chicken breast, creating a pocket. Add enough tomato mixture to fill each pocket and transfer the chicken to a baking sheet.

▸ Bake for about 15 minutes, until the chicken juices run clear. Top with any remaining stuffing.

▸ While chicken is cooking, sauté the spinach with the remaining Tbsp of olive oil and minced garlic clove. Serve alongside the chicken.

MAKES 2 SERVINGS.

Meal Maker
Eat with ½ cup of potatoes.

NUTRITION PER SERVING
634 CALORIES | 60 G PROTEIN | 29 G CARBOHYDRATES (2 G FIBER) | 29 G FAT

MH BEST MEALS FOR MUSCLE

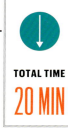

TOTAL TIME
20 MIN

PAPRIKA CHICKEN
with Crispy Chickpeas and Tomatoes

WHAT YOU'LL NEED

- 12 OZ TOMATOES
- 8 CLOVES GARLIC, SMASHED, IN THEIR SKINS
- 1 (15-oz) CAN CHICKPEAS, RINSED
- 3 TBSP OLIVE OIL, DIVIDED
- KOSHER SALT AND PEPPER
- 4 (6-OZ) BONELESS, SKINLESS CHICKEN BREASTS
- 2 TSP PAPRIKA

HOW TO MAKE IT

▶ Heat oven to 425°F. On a rimmed baking sheet, toss tomatoes, garlic and chickpeas with 2 Tbsp oil and ¼ tsp each salt and pepper. Roast 10 minutes.

▶ Heat remaining Tbsp oil in large skillet on medium. Season chicken with paprika and ½ tsp each salt and pepper and cook until golden brown on one side, 5 to 6 minutes. Flip and cook 1 minute more. Transfer to baking sheet with tomatoes and chickpeas and roast until cooked through, 6 minutes more. Before serving, discard garlic skins.

MAKES 4 SERVINGS.

Meal Maker
Eat with 1 cup of potatoes.

NUTRITION PER SERVING
390 CALORIES | 40 G PROTEIN | 21 G CARBOHYDRATES (6 G FIBER) | 16 G FAT

DINNER

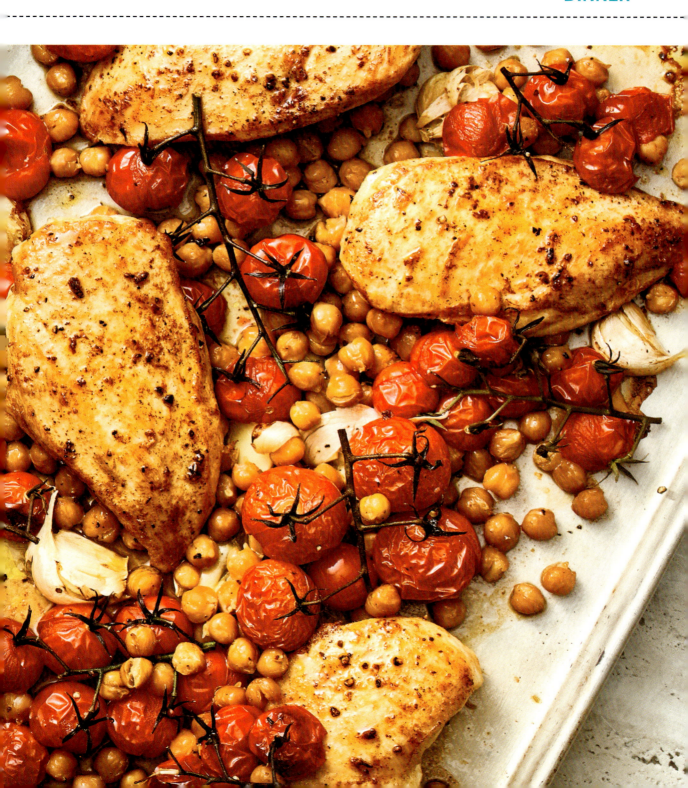

MH BEST MEALS FOR MUSCLE

HERBED MOJO STEAK AND CRISPY POTATOES

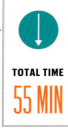

TOTAL TIME
55 MIN

WHAT YOU'LL NEED

- 3 CLOVES GARLIC, GRATED
- 1 SMALL RED CHILE, THINLY SLICED
- ⅓ CUP FLAT-LEAF PARSLEY
- ⅓ CUP FRESH CILANTRO
- ⅓ CUP FRESH BASIL
- 2 TBSP LIME JUICE
- 2 TBSP ORANGE JUICE, PLUS WEDGES FOR SERVING
- ¼ TSP GROUND CUMIN
- ¼ CUP OLIVE OIL, DIVIDED
- KOSHER SALT AND GROUND BLACK PEPPER
- 2 1-IN.-THICK STRIP STEAKS (about 1½ lbs total)
- 2 SMALL RED ONIONS, CUT INTO ½-IN.-THICK WEDGES
- 4 SMALL YELLOW POTATOES (about 1¼ lbs), CUT INTO ¾-IN.-THICK WEDGES

HOW TO MAKE IT

- In a blender, puree garlic, chile, parsley, cilantro, basil, lime juice, orange juice, cumin, 2 Tbsp olive oil, and ¼ tsp salt until smooth.

- Transfer ¼ cup of mixture to a shallow dish and add beef, turning to coat (reserve remaining sauce for serving). Let sit for 15 minutes.

- Meanwhile, preheat the oven to 425°F. Grease a large rimmed baking sheet with 1 Tbsp oil. Arrange onions and potatoes on sheet, season with ½ tsp each salt and pepper, and roast until golden brown and tender, 20 to 25 minutes.

- Heat remaining Tbsp oil in a large skillet on medium. Season beef with ¼ tsp each salt and pepper and cook until browned and to desired doneness, 8 to 9 minutes per side for medium-rare. Serve with vegetables, reserved sauce, and orange wedges for squeezing.

MAKES 4 SERVINGS.

Meal Maker
Eat with 1 cup of vegetables.

NUTRITION PER SERVING
530 CALORIES | 26 G FAT | 39 G PROTEIN | 36 G CARBOHYDRATES (5 G FIBER)

DINNER

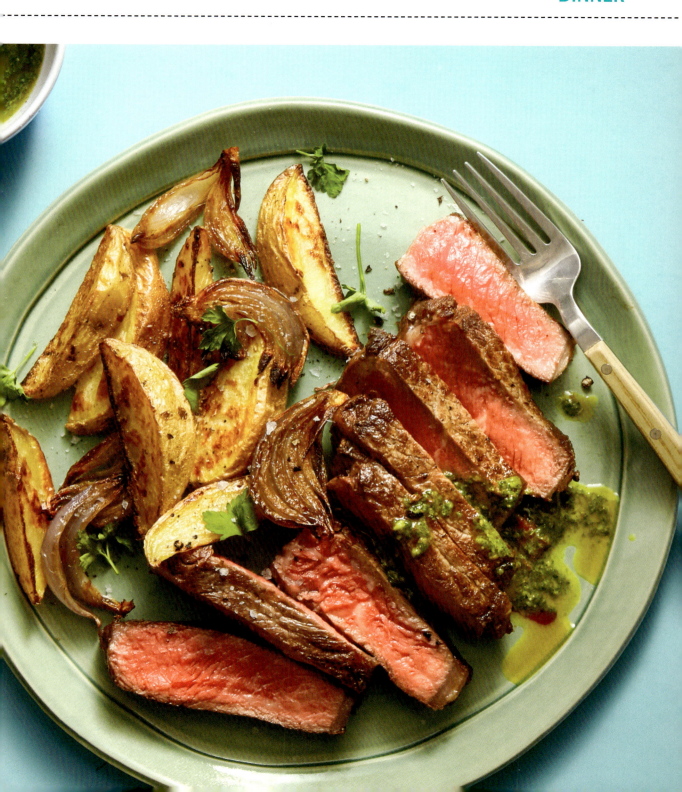

MH BEST MEALS FOR MUSCLE

TOTAL TIME
35 MIN

SHEET PAN CHICKPEA CHICKEN

WHAT YOU'LL NEED

- 1 (15.5-oz) CAN CHICKPEAS, RINSED
- 1 (16-oz) BAG MINI SWEET PEPPERS
- 2 TBSP HARISSA SAUCE
- 4 SMALL SKIN-ON CHICKEN LEGS (about 2½ lbs)

CHOPPED CILANTRO, FOR SERVING

HOW TO MAKE IT

- Preheat the oven to 425°F. On a large rimmed baking sheet, toss chickpeas and peppers with 1 Tbsp oil, ¼ tsp each salt and pepper.

- In a small bowl, whisk together harissa and 1 Tbsp oil. Rub chicken with harissa mixture. Nestle among chickpeas and peppers and roast until chicken is golden brown and cooked through, 20 to 25 minutes.

- Toss with cilantro before serving.

MAKES 4 SERVINGS.

Meal Maker
Eat with ½ cup of brown rice.

NUTRITION PER SERVING
630 CALORIES | 39 G PROTEIN | 22 G CARBOHYDRATES (6 G FIBER) | 42 G FAT

DINNER

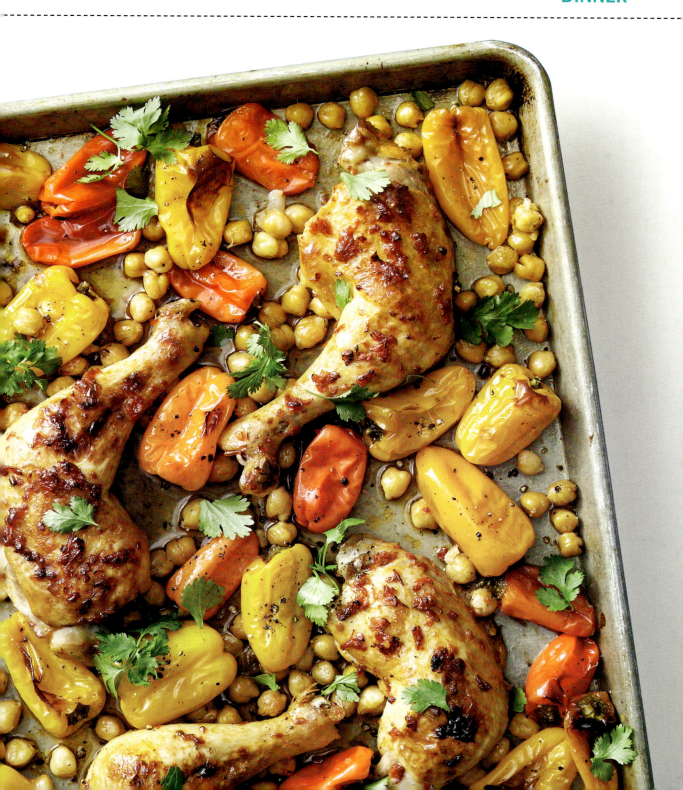

MH BEST MEALS FOR MUSCLE

CHILI MANGO CHICKEN

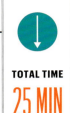

TOTAL TIME
25 MIN

WHAT YOU'LL NEED

- 1 LB BONELESS, SKINLESS CHICKEN THIGHS, CUT INTO ½-IN. PIECES
- 1 TBSP CORNSTARCH
- 1 TBSP LOWER SODIUM SOY SAUCE
- 1½ TSP SESAME OIL
- 1½ TSP PEANUT OR CANOLA OIL
- 1 RED ONION, CHOPPED
- 1 TBSP GRATED OR MINCED FRESH GINGER
- 2 CUPS SUGAR SNAP PEAS
- 1 MANGO, CHOPPED
- 1 TBSP CHILI GARLIC SAUCE, PREFERABLY HUY FONG
- GROUND BLACK PEPPER

HOW TO MAKE IT

▶ In a large bowl, combine the chicken, cornstarch, soy sauce, and sesame oil and let it sit for 10 minutes.

▶ Heat the peanut or canola oil in a wok or large skillet over high heat. Add the onion and ginger and cook until the onion is translucent, 1 to 2 minutes. Add the peas and stir-fry for 1 minute. Add the chicken with its marinade and stir-fry until it begins to brown, about 2 minutes.

▶ Add the mango, chili garlic sauce, and black pepper to taste. Stir-fry until the chicken is cooked through and the mango becomes saucy, about 1 minute more.

MAKES 4 SERVINGS.

Meal Maker
Eat with 1 cup brown rice.

 NUTRITION PER SERVING
355 CALORIES | 32 G PROTEIN | 19 G CARBOHYDRATES (3 G FIBER) | 16 G FAT

DINNER

SWEET AND SOUR PORK

TOTAL TIME
35 MIN

WHAT YOU'LL NEED

- 2 TBSP SOY SAUCE
- 4 TSP RICE WINE OR DRY SHERRY
- 1 TSP SESAME OIL
- ¼ TSP COARSE SALT
- ¼ TSP GROUND BLACK PEPPER
- ½ TSP + 2 TBSP SUGAR, DIVIDED
- 1 LB PORK BUTT OR SHOULDER, FAT TRIMMED, CUT INTO 1-IN. CUBES
- ½ CUP ALL-PURPOSE FLOUR
- ½ CUP + 1 TBSP CORNSTARCH, DIVIDED
- 1 (20-oz) CAN JUICE-PACKED PINEAPPLE CHUNKS
- ⅓ CUP KETCHUP
- ⅓ CUP DISTILLED WHITE VINEGAR
- 1 CUP + 1 TBSP PEANUT OIL OR OTHER VEGETABLE OIL, DIVIDED
- 4 SLICES FRESH GINGER
- 1 GREEN BELL PEPPER, CUT INTO 1-IN. SQUARES

HOW TO MAKE IT

▶ In a large bowl, combine the soy sauce, rice wine or sherry, sesame oil, salt, pepper, and ½ tsp of the sugar. Add the pork, toss to coat, and marinate 10 minutes.

▶ In another bowl, combine the flour and ½ cup of the cornstarch. Drain the pork, reserving the marinade. Lightly dredge the pork pieces in the flour-cornstarch mixture and set them aside on a plate.

▶ Drain the pineapple chunks, reserving ½ cup of the juice. Add the juice to the bowl of reserved marinade and stir in the ketchup, vinegar, and remaining 2 Tbsp sugar and 1 Tbsp cornstarch.

▶ Heat 1 cup of the oil in a 14-in. flat-bottomed wok until it's hot but not smoking. Add half the pork, spreading the pieces around in the oil. Cook 1 to 2 minutes until they begin to brown and then turn them. After 3 to 4 minutes, when the pieces are browned on all sides, transfer them to a plate lined with a paper towel. Repeat with the rest of the pork.

▶ Rinse and dry the wok, and return it to high heat. Add the remaining 1 Tbsp oil and the ginger and stir-fry 10 seconds. Add the green pepper and stir-fry 1 minute. Add the reserved pineapple chunks and swirl the sweet-and-sour sauce into the wok. Bring the mixture to a boil, stirring until it's just thickened, about 1 minute. Add the pork and cook, stirring, for 2 to 3 minutes.

MAKES 4 SERVINGS.

NUTRITION PER SERVING
498 CALORIES | 24 G PROTEIN | 40 G CARBOHYDRATES (2 G FIBER) | 26 G FAT

MH BEST MEALS FOR MUSCLE

FRESH VEGGIE BEEF RAGU

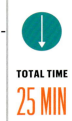

TOTAL TIME
25 MIN

WHAT YOU'LL NEED

- 12 OZ LINGUINE
- 1 LEMON
- 2 TBSP OIL
- 1 LB LEAN GROUND BEEF
- 2 CLOVES GARLIC
- 2 TBSP TOMATO PASTE
- ½ CUP DRY WHITE WINE
- 1 PT CHERRY TOMATOES
- ½ RED ONION
- PARMESAN AND BASIL, IF DESIRED

HOW TO MAKE IT

- Cook linguine according to package directions. Before draining, reserve 1 cup cooking liquid and set aside. Drain and return pasta to pot.
- Grate the zest from the lemon directly into the pot. Then squeeze in the lemon juice.
- Add 1 Tbsp oil, and toss pasta together. Add reserved cooking liquid if the pasta seems dry.
- While the pasta cooks, brown ground beef in a large skillet in 1 Tbsp oil, breaking it up into tiny pieces, 6 minutes.
- Finely chop garlic and stir into pasta; cook 1 minute.
- Add tomato paste and cook, stirring, until beef starts to get crispy.
- Add dry white wine and simmer until it evaporates, 3 minutes.
- Thinly slice red onion. Cut cherry tomatoes in half.
- Toss the beef with pasta, cherry tomatoes, and red onion. Sprinkle with Parmesan and basil if desired.

MAKES 4 SERVINGS.

NUTRITION PER SERVING
545 CALORIES | 36 G PROTEIN | 72 G CARB (5 G FIBER) | 14 G FAT

DINNER

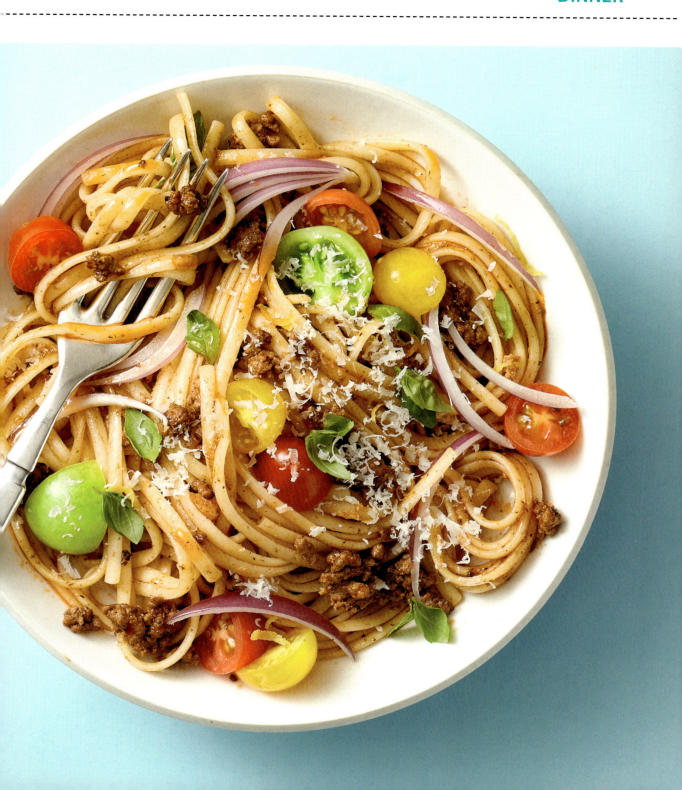

MH BEST MEALS FOR MUSCLE

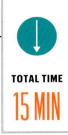

TOTAL TIME
15 MIN

SALMON TERIYAKI
With Asparagus

WHAT YOU'LL NEED

- 2 TBSP LOWER SODIUM SOY SAUCE
- 2 TBSP MIRIN
- 1 TBSP HONEY
- 1 TBSP CHILI GARLIC SAUCE, SUCH AS SRIRACHA
- 1 TSP CORNSTARCH
- 1 TSP SESAME OIL
- 1 TBSP MINCED FRESH GINGER
- 2 CLOVES GARLIC, FINELY CHOPPED
- 1 TBSP VEGETABLE OIL, PREFERABLY PEANUT
- 1 LB SKINLESS SALMON, CUT INTO 1-IN. CUBES
- 1 BUNCH ASPARAGUS, CUT INTO THIRDS
- 1 TBSP SESAME SEEDS (optional)

HOW TO MAKE IT

▶ In a small bowl, whisk together the soy sauce, mirin, honey, chili garlic sauce, cornstarch, sesame oil, ginger, and garlic. Set the mixture aside.

▶ Heat a wok or large skillet over medium-high heat. When it's hot, add the vegetable oil and swirl to coat the pan. Add the salmon pieces and cook, stirring occasionally, until they just begin to turn opaque, about 2 minutes. Transfer them to a plate.

▶ Add the asparagus to the wok and stir-fry until crisp-tender, about 2 minutes. Return the salmon to the wok and stir in the soy sauce mixture. Heat, stirring, for 1 minute. If the sauce seems too thick, add a couple of Tbsp of water. Garnish with sesame seeds.

MAKES 4 SERVINGS.

Meal Maker
Eat with 1 cup brown rice.

NUTRITION PER SERVING
379 CALORIES | 31 G PROTEIN | 35 G CARBOHYDRATES (5 G FIBER) | 12 G FAT

DINNER

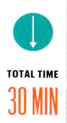

TOTAL TIME
30 MIN

SMOKY AND SPICY SAUSAGE HEROES

WHAT YOU'LL NEED

- 1 TBSP EXTRA-VIRGIN OLIVE OIL
- 1 LB SMOKED TURKEY SAUSAGE
- 1 RED BELL PEPPER, THINLY SLICED
- ½ ONION, THINLY SLICED
- 2 (8-in.) WHOLE WHEAT SUB OR HERO ROLLS
- ½ CUP ARUGULA
- HOT SAUCE

HOW TO MAKE IT

▶ Heat the oil in a large, heavy skillet over medium heat until it shimmers. Add the sausage and cover the pan. Cook, turning the sausage links occasionally, until they're browned and cooked through, 10 to 12 minutes.

▶ Remove the sausage from the pan and set aside. Add the pepper and onion and cook, stirring occasionally, until softened, about 8 minutes. Return the sausages to the pan and cook until hot, 1 to 2 minutes.

▶ While the sausage is cooking, split and toast the rolls. When everything's ready, fill each roll with a piece of sausage and some pepper-onion mixture and arugula. Add hot sauce to taste.

MAKES 2 SERVINGS.

NUTRITION PER SERVING

618 CALORIES | 41 G PROTEIN | 58 G CARBOHYDRATES (9 G FIBER) | 26 G FAT

BEST MEALS FOR MUSCLE

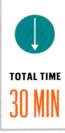

TOTAL TIME
30 MIN

SPICED MEATBALL PITAS
with Crispy Cole Slaw

WHAT YOU'LL NEED

- 1 LB GROUND LAMB OR BEEF
- 2 TSP SMOKED PAPRIKA
- 1 TSP GROUND CORIANDER
- ½ TSP SALT
- ½ LB LARGER CARROTS, PEELED
- 1 (2-in.) PIECE GINGER, PEELED
- CILANTRO, TO TASTE
- 4 PITAS
- ½ CUP GREEK YOGURT
- 2 TSP HARISSA

HOW TO MAKE IT

▶ In a bowl, combine meat, paprika, coriander, and salt. Roll into 1-in. bars (about 35) and arrange on nonstick foil-rimmed baking sheet. Broil until cooked through, 6 to 8 min.

▶ Coarsely grate the carrots and ginger. Heat oil in large skillet on medium-high and fry carrots and ginger, in batches, until crisp, 3 to 5 minutes; transfer to paper towels to drain, then toss with cilantro.

▶ Stuff halved pitas with meatballs and carrot slaw and drizzle with mixture of ½ cup Greek yogurt and 2 tsp harissa.

MAKES 4 SERVINGS.

Meal Maker
Eat with 1 cup vegetables.

 NUTRITION PER SERVING | 505 CALORIES | 28 G PROTEIN | 42 G CARBOHYDRATES (3 G FIBER) | 24.5 G FAT

DINNER

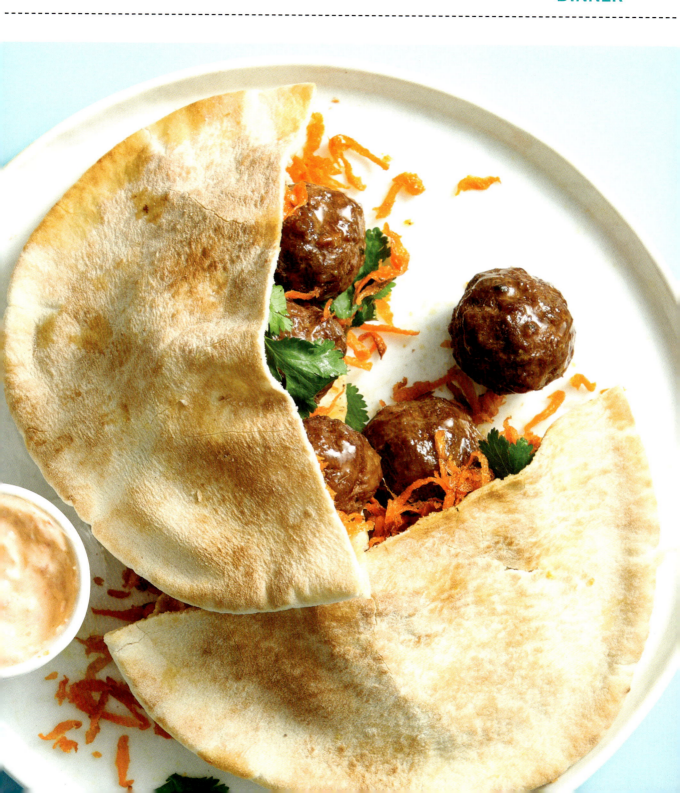

THANK YOU
FOR PURCHASING BEST MEALS FOR MUSCLE

Boost your fitness with more from *Men's Health*!
Visit our online store and
save 20% off your first purchase.

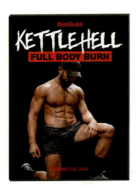 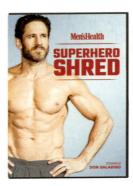 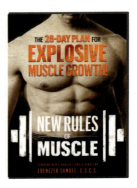

PLEASE ENJOY 20% OFF AT OUR STORE!

20% OFF
USE COUPON CODE THANKYOU20

Shop.MensHealth.com

Offer only applies to books, guides, DVDs, and new magazine subscription purchases and is not eligible on Airbnb and Pioneer Woman Magazine. This discount is not redeemable in combination with other promotions; additional restrictions may apply.